A STROKE OF GENIUS

To Tom and Cheryl
You've been there!
Carpé diem —

Sandy Sorrin
1/9/02

A
Message

"This is an account of a very personal journey, a journey that starts with... a cerebral hemorrhage. It leads through paths of paralysis and pain to healing and new insight into the nature of the human condition. Nothing could be more devastating than a severe stroke. The greatest fear for many of us is that we should survive... and be severely limited in our ability to communicate, move and live independently. Sandy Simon tells us how he dealt with this experience and developed a much broader range of perceptions and sensitivities as a consequence. His story is about the power of courage, humor and the support of other human beings. There are valuable lessons here for each of us."

Dr. Peter Doherty
Nobel Laureate
at St. Jude Children's Research Hospital
Memphis, Tennessee

A STROKE OF GENIUS

MESSAGES OF HOPE AND HEALING FROM A THRIVING STROKE SURVIVOR

Sandy Simon

The Cedars Group
Delray Beach, Florida
2001

Library of Congress Control Number: 2001118304

ISBN 0-9669625-2-4

Printed in the United States of America

Dedicated
to
my physical therapist and friend

Rebecca

and to all therapists everywhere who enable so many of
us stroke survivors to rebuild our lives. To the
paramedics, EMTs, and the medical profession to
whom I am most grateful for their dedication, training,
counsel, and continued efforts to improve the lives of
stroke victims everywhere.

Acknowledgements

I am grateful to Christiane for her friendship, support, and collaboration in helping me share my story and its messages. She was my researcher, my typist, my organizer and, in many ways, my editor. Her encouragement during those emotionally difficult days helped me overcome and continue.

I am also grateful to my family and friends who encouraged me to write this book and to Jean Goode who professionally guided me through my literary endeavors.

Table of Contents

Preface

I wrote this book after a six-year odyssey following a stroke, a severe cerebral hemorrhage that came within an hour of causing either my death or complete emotional, mental and physical incapacity. I found a way to healing and thriving as a human being and have achieved a new peace and improved life of joy, happiness and serenity.

A Stroke of Genius is written to help people who have suffered and survived a stroke, their caregivers, loved ones, family, colleagues, friends and therapists everywhere.

Many stroke victims may not even want to continue living after their stroke, but this book should help them see a brighter future in spite of their impairments and help them learn to enjoy a new life more than they ever thought possible.

Sandy Simon

Foreword

Sandy Simon's book, *A STROKE OF GENIUS*, should be required reading for everyone. As a neurologist specializing in acute stroke treatment, I urge all doctors, neurologists, therapists and caregivers to **READ THIS BOOK!**

It is essential for all medical students, nurses and physicians who deal with stroke patients. I have read many books and studies on stroke, and this is the best I've seen. It offers powerful insight into the stroke survivor's mind, that guide the reader to discover the path to healing physically, emotionally and attitudinally. It clearly, easily, and sometimes humorously conveys the message that healing after a stroke and once again returning to a thriving, productive and meaningful lifestyle requires total treatment.

Severe crisis by itself is merely pain, but the experience of pain, coupled with the understanding that the pain can serve a worthy purpose can constitute meaningful suffering. Sandy Simon shows us that seeking out with courage and bringing into the Light of Consciousness that which is unconscious is the path to healing.

Mr. Simon makes a solid case that faith, attitude, tenacity and interaction with caregivers and loved ones is the most meaningful solution to the devastation of this terrible affliction.

Dr. Mark L. Brody,
Neurologist and Stroke Specialist
Medical Director, Bethesda Hospital Stroke Program
Florida International University, Miami, Florida

Introduction

When Mr. Simon asked me to consider writing an introduction to his book, I immediately agreed to do so. After all, he was a friend of a friend.

I prepared myself to write some saccharine-sweet comments to indulge the author of a saccharine-sweet book about the recovery from a stroke.

Then I read the manuscript, and now I plead guilty to the possession of an ill-informed and condescending attitude.

As a physical therapist and professor of physical therapy, I already have knowledge about stroke and stroke rehabilitation. What I found so useful in Mr. Simon's book is the opportunity to gain *wisdom* about stroke and stroke rehabilitation.

Mr. Simon has written from a unique perspective; he describes the process of stroke rehabilitation from the patient's perspective. We therapists are so undereducated when it comes to understanding the impact of our therapies on the whole person, and Mr. Simon's memories, anecdotes, and insights are enlightening. How useful the book would have been to me if I had read it before I worked with my first patient some 25 years ago.

My experience as a therapist has been that recovery after stroke is strongly influenced by some intangible quality that exists almost independently of the medical condition. It is this intangible quality, which grows out of a combination of attitude, faith, motivation, and interactions with friends and family that Mr. Simon so clearly understands and articulates.

Leonard Elbaum, EdD, PT
Associate Professor of Physical Therapy
Florida International University, Miami, Florida

Chapter 1

My Story

On Sunday evening November 28, 1993, five days after my 56th birthday, I awakened from a nap on my bed at 5 p.m. to shower for a dinner engagement. When I tried to lift myself up, my left arm collapsed. That's weird, what is this? I asked myself about this strange failure of my left side. I was not yet aware that my entire left side was totally numb, unfeeling, and paralyzed. I rolled onto my left side, and, thinking both my legs had slid out from under the cover as I thought I had instructed them, I shifted my weight. Unknown to me, my numb left hip was off the edge of the bed, my left leg and foot got caught in the bed sheet, and I clumsily fell off the bed onto the floor. What's happening? I thought, frightened. I was aware that something very strange was happening to me, but I had no idea what it was. I tried to stand up and crashed into my armoire, face first. Then, I fell again onto the floor, my face striking a wastebasket. What the hell is going on? I had fallen down three times. I remember becoming really alarmed. I was alone in my home and began feeling very alone physically *and* emotionally. I thought that maybe I was having a bad dream. Nervously, I crawled slowly toward the bed, which was just a few feet away. I couldn't believe what was happening. I had no power, no control. My left arm was flopping and my left leg was also totally lifeless. I grabbed the bed clothing and pulled myself back onto the bed using all my strength pulling with my right arm and pushing my right leg while dragging my left side.

Dripping with perspiration, I was absolutely terrified and trying to figure out what was going on. Many thoughts raced through my mind. Strangely, I had no pain and no chest constriction, none whatsoever. It didn't feel like a heart attack. My heart was racing with fear. I remember asking myself time and again, What could this be? Could it be a stroke?

Like most people in America in 1993, I knew next to nothing about strokes. So little was in the public consciousness. Most media coverage at the time was devoted to AIDS, its cure and its national fundraising efforts, or with cancer. So little was known about the brain. The American Heart Association did not even create its American Stroke Association as a new division until 1997 and the National Stroke Association was established as recently as 1984.

The only experience I ever had with stroke was with my father who over a number of years suffered a series of transient ischemic attacks (TIAs). Eventually, my father died of pneumonia in 1979 at the age of 77, from complications resulting from those strokes. "Hardening of the arteries" was the labeled culprit. That description always sounded so untreatable to me, so final, so terminal. I watched my father, a giant in my life, brought down by a series of strokes to a weakened, crippled man who was unable to stand, walk, use his hands or legs, or speak well. I knew he was given lots of medication, mostly palliatives. That is about all the treatment he had besides a rubber ball to squeeze with his hands, and several infrequent visits by a sympathetic therapist. I watched him consume an abundance of prescribed capsules and pills during my caregiver visits from Atlanta those last years. He was seemingly "doped up" all the time by the drugs. I was with him often, and watched with great sadness as he got weaker and weaker, unable to control his bodily functions, having to be cared for completely everyday by my 75-year-old mother and her 77-year-old sister. He could not walk without assistance. He couldn't bathe himself. He was incontinent and he could not keep his balance. My mother and her sister had to nearly carry my father from the living room, where he spent most of his days, to the bathroom. Then, with great embarrassment to him I am sure, they bathed him in the shower as he sat on a chair.

He became very lethargic and completely different from his former self. His personality changed significantly. He had no self-confidence, no energy. Some days he seemed to have resigned himself to his hopeless fate. The worst part was that he was aware of his condition and how difficult it was for everyone he loved and who loved him. He was trapped in a body that could no longer function.

These memories became painfully vivid to me as I experienced this awful and sudden attack on my body. I began to realize that, like my father, I might lose *my* capabilities. And I believed if this was in fact a stroke, I would be incapacitated for the rest of *my* life. And I became aware that like my father, my future might be over. I was terrified at the prospect of being unable to care for myself for years and years. I was, after all, only 56 years old. I remember crying as I thought about my father, DEAR GOD, NOT A STROKE. ANYTHING BUT A STROKE! OH GOD, PLEASE, PLEASE, PLEASE NOT A STROKE.

My fear of stroke was not a fear of death but of the permanent disabilities. That is what frightened me so much when I began to realize that I might indeed be suffering a stroke.

There was no warning. Every second that went by became more and more urgent, more frightening, and I became aware more and more that I was very much alone. I remember asking myself, and maybe I asked God too, Is this it? Is this how it happens? I didn't think that I was dying but if I was, I was OK with that. Interestingly, I think at that moment I preferred to die rather than suffer a severe, life-changing, crippling stroke. And then I realized it was up to me to do something. I quickly reached across my body with my right hand, grabbed the phone and called for help.

I called my brother Roy and, I remember, explained, "Roy, something terrible has happened. I think I've had a stroke and I need help, please." Weeks later, Roy told me he sensed an emergency when he heard a bunch of garbling, slurring, nonsensical gobbledygook and could only recognize my voice. He said to me, which I heard clearly, "I'll be right over. Call 911. So will I." I still remember my exact words and his. I also remember dialing 911, hearing the woman's voice, and explaining the same thing to her as I told my brother. She said to me, "Can you speak English?" I think I laughed and replied, "Speak English? I've never been asked that in South Florida." I thought that was very funny since Spanish, Haitian and 98 other dialects are now spoken in South Florida, including various forms of broken English. But she came through for me, and the system worked perfectly in my favor. I was lucky it did! I suppose, like Roy, all she heard were slurred, unintelligible sounds, not words.

Actually, the emergency people (EMT) arrived after Roy, and while I talked to him, frantically and in gibberish I'm sure, the EMT tried to calm me down while they put an oxygen mask on my face and whatever else they do. But I began to feel safe as they cared for me, and I could see my brother's face and feel his touch. I remember the last thing I saw and heard was the paramedic placing the oxygen mask on my face as he reassured me, "You're going to be OK...we're here now. You're going to be fine." I also remember thinking, Thank you God for sending Roy and the emergency rescue people. Then I slipped off into la-la land where I apparently stayed for several days.

I was placed in intensive care at Bethesda Hospital, where for five days I underwent four CT scans, MRIs, multiple tests and examinations. I had suffered a cerebrovascular accident (CVA). Specifically, my diagnosis was a cerebral hemorrhage, one of the two main types of stroke, which was caused by a burst blood vessel in my brain. I was unconscious the whole time, thank God, and didn't know about the tubes down my throat, the IV's and the tests. I was the star of this horror production, but my "lights were out."

I was then sent to Pinecrest Rehabilitation Hospital a few miles away. There, by the luck of the draw, I became a patient of Rebecca Reubens, physical therapist, and Kerry Brown, occupational therapist, two of the best therapists at Pinecrest in my opinion. Later, I learned that therapists there, maybe everywhere, are assigned certain beds and whoever is given that bed becomes their patient.

I stayed there for three days suffering excruciatingly painful headaches. My relatives who visited me tell me that my eyes were closed as I pointed to my right temple where my head hurt so much. I also suffered from non-stop hiccups that relentlessly shook my body and interrupted every thought process.

The doctors gave me injections of Thorazine to stop the hiccups. One day when my dear friends from high school, Tom Butts, then living in North Carolina, and Richard Machek, came to visit me, I told them about the hiccups and Thorazine injections. Tom said, "We give that to our horses to settle them down when they get over-excited. That'll sure stop hiccups 'cause you are a lot smaller than a horse, Sandy." And sure enough, the hiccups stopped. That Thorazine sure did calm me down! I couldn't open my eyes for nearly a month. Talk about relaxed!

In early December, after my second day in therapy, Rebecca saved my life. She had become alarmed at my sudden and rapidly deteriorating condition. She convinced my brothers and doctors that I was failing fast, that I could not make the next 48 hours without emergency care. They responded and immediately transferred me back to Bethesda Hospital's Intensive Care Unit. More tests, MRIs and CT scans showed unexpected rapidly growing pressure due to severe fluid penetration into my left brain from the right side of my brain, which made the midline of my brain press against my left skull. My *entire* brain was virtually being squeezed to death by the pressure. There was a dual threat and a question of whether the pressure from the extreme bleeding would destroy my left brain before it reached my brain stem. My neurologist and doctors had three options: wait and see, drill or give me heavy doses of diuretics. The best thing would have been to remove the top of my skull until the swelling went down, but that of course was not an option. They made their decision: I was treated medically with diuretics to relieve the pressure. The doctors decided not to drill because the blood vessel was too deep. The right side of my brain was already severely damaged. Further damage to the left side would have killed me. For some wonderful reason, my bleeding stopped within that hour.

I was returned by ambulance to Pinecrest Rehab Hospital on December 9th. For two weeks I was in a serious, semi-comatose condition. My friends came. My brothers came. I could hear them speak to me. I could understand them very well. And I thought I was speaking clearly to them in return, always with my eyes closed. But later I was told that I spoke very slowly with slurred speech and with garbled, unintelligible sounds. I had trouble speaking too because of those incessant hiccups.

It was a traumatically difficult time for those closest to me who loved me as I loved them. They were given very little hope. At first, the doctors' messages were: "He's had a very severe attack on his brain. He has had an artery in his brain explode deep in the right side behind his ear. The damage is severe and massive." (I live with the physical results to this day.) "We know so little about the brain, we cannot tell you what his condition will be. But it's bad. Very bad. We'll just have to wait and see. No two strokes are alike." My family — my brothers Ernie, Roy and Charlie, and my dear cousins Zicky, Dudley, Rodney and Nancy — could see I was in a terrible, seemingly hopeless, shape in the hospital bed. They could tell I was in severe pain and completely immobile. I constantly hiccuped and was hydrated from those familiar clear plastic bags filled with some fluid that hung from stainless steel standing poles. Clear plastic tubes ran downward from the bottom of these bags taped to the bed rail and were finally connected to the shunt in my hand where I received the welcomed fluids into my body.

They came and went daily after visiting me during what turned out to be a very depressing vigil for them. Someone had to assume the dreaded responsibilities of what to do with me if I died...what to do with me if I didn't die...how to handle my affairs, my business...what to do with their 56-year-old brother who was vibrant one day and struck down so suddenly, so cruelly the next. Maybe they would have to find a way for me to be cared for twenty-four hours a day for many years. Who knew? They had no idea what the next moment held, much less the next day. They had only what the doctors and nurses would tell them which was frustratingly indefinite. And the doctors only knew what they interpreted from the frightening results of the many CT scans and MRIs that had been taken of my brain, which showed such massive damages that no one would venture an optimistic prognosis. *"If he doesn't live...if he lives..."* My family and I felt frustration because we both knew they couldn't really help me. They could only convey their love and their encouragement. I wanted to be with them instead of trapped in this broken body lying in bed unable to move.

No one had any reason to believe I would actually survive, even my cousin Dr. Neil Zane, my personal physician, later told me, "Sandy, your damage was so great that I decided I would never want you to see your MRIs and CT scans. You would be so depressed, you might just give up." It seemed there was no reason for hope by anyone in my world. That is what the neurologists believed, what the radiologists *knew*, and what the doctors *knew*. They actually believed there was very little reason for hope. Their reality was a horror story about my life.

So, while I was lucky enough not to know the severity of my damage, my most loved ones were not spared the news and had to brace themselves for the worst. And that is something we stroke victims must remind ourselves: that our loved ones and supporters have to carry a heavy emotional load that may, in some ways, be heavier than we, the patients, have to bear. And that includes the time long after we leave the hospital. Yet, we are so consumed with our own situation, self-pity and self-concern that we don't have much emotional room for our caregivers' feelings. Now, in retrospect, I know we should.

During the early portion of my hospital stay, I did very little fantasizing, perceiving, envisioning or encouraging. I actually did little but sleep, rest, and eat whatever someone put into my mouth. And lots of people did just that I've been told. I must have been very trusting during my semi-comatose days, because so many people have since told me, "I fed you lunch," or "I fed you dinner. It was so sad having to feed you Sandy." But I felt happiness each time a dear friend told me that. For a long time, I cried, "How did this happen? What happened to my body? I am trapped in this crippled body and I can't get out." I was miserable.

After the initial three weeks, I slowly began the cycle of grief: denial, depression, anger, bargaining, and acceptance. I recycled those emotions in my mind hundreds of times. I also began that day to determine that I had to change my perception of life, develop a new response and new determination and muster all the courage God would give me. As I spoke with dear friends and my brothers, I slowly began to develop a new attitude, a new perception. I still had trouble with the emotional roller coaster of the cycle of grief...I would sometimes cry at the slightest impulse...seeing a visitor for whom I cared very much...a glance at my left arm hanging there lifeless...an old friend with a smile. It was an awful time, so sad, and so depressing.

A total lack of confidence...a complete loss of self-esteem...my emotions were on a roller coaster ride...up then down...up then down...rarely stable.

As I lay in my hospital bed, I concentrated all day on my life before the stroke. I had become so filled with a sense of guilt (part of the post-stroke syndrome) that I remembered every past personal and business relationship in great detail. I remembered everything I'd ever done that may have hurt someone and felt great disappointment in myself. My greatest worry was what would happen to me now. Would I be like this the rest of my life...helpless, unable to feed or bathe myself, confined to a wheelchair? How would I live? When I asked the doctors, the answer always was: "We don't know...we just don't know. No two strokes are alike." There seemed little medical reason for hope. They were convinced that I would become a physical, mental and emotional invalid. I wallowed in self-pity and there were times when I thought that those who died were lucky.

Even so, I held onto my faith in God. I hoped that the doctors could be wrong and that I would be healed and walk again, that I would drive again and make decisions again. Walking and driving meant independence and a sense of freedom. I made a total commitment to my healing. I completely obeyed my therapists' instructions. For hours I exercised my mouth, my face, my tongue, my leg. I was thrilled when I moved my big toe, slightly. But it moved! It was all I could move at first. My left arm wouldn't respond, as it turned out, for five months.

I've been told that many people came to see me after the first few weeks when I was "out of it." I would somehow tell jokes as my speech began to return. My favorite was, "It's eleven o'clock. Does anybody know where my left leg is?" I would laugh and talk about friendships, always with my eyes closed, and pointing at my head because of the severe headaches.

On December 20th, nearly one month after the stroke, Kerry, my occupational therapist, tested my visual ability and cognitive capabilities. She asked me to draw a picture of myself, and then to copy pictures of a clock, a daisy, and a house. My drawing of myself showed no left arm, left leg, left ear or left eye. My copies of the clock had no number seven through eleven and the daisy had no petals on the left side. The house had no windows, chimney or roofline on the left — the entire left side was missing — and I was a trained architectural engineer! I thought the drawings were perfect! Of course they weren't. A month later I drew another set and compared the two. Here was verification in black and white. I could no longer deny the damage. It was clear that it went beyond my left leg and arm. Not only could I not see to my left, I couldn't conceive the left, and I didn't even know it.

A very exciting moment for me was on Christmas Eve. I was in my fifth week in the hospital, having a melancholy day. All of a sudden I heard a familiar voice singing. Then I heard two familiar voices singing down the corridor. The voices kept getting a little louder as the two men walked toward my room. They were singing Christmas carols. As their voices became very clear, I looked to the door. Standing in the doorway singing, "I'll be home for Christmas..." were my dear friends Tony Butala, lead singer of The Lettermen, and my cousin Zicky, another fine singer. I couldn't believe it. What an honor! Tony and The Lettermen were appearing in the nearby town of Jupiter and my dear cousin Helen had called Tony. He took time from his very busy schedule at 6 p.m. on Christmas Eve to come see me. I was stunned and cried tears of joy. It was a moment I will never forget. I was so inspired that after they left I tried to get out of my wheelchair to take a shower. Of course, I crashed on the bathroom floor, cracked my head, and bled all over the place. Tony and Zicky's visit must have convinced me I could actually shower, dress and go to church. But of course I couldn't. I just believed I could. Their visit meant so much to me; my relevance to the world was still possible, and that was a great inspiration for me to get well.

During my third month at Pinecrest, I was given a comprehensive series of psycho-neurological tests, some of which were like SAT tests. They were meant to determine what parts of my brain had survived. They tested motor functions, information processing, long and short term memory, deductive reasoning, behavioral relationships, language comprehension and usage, mental flexibility and fluency, visual and spatial analysis, English and math. I was amazed to learn that I scored above the 94th percentile. I am sure I scored higher on those SAT tests than I would have before the stroke. And since my grade was based on U.S. standards of those tested with or without brain damage in the 40-60 age bracket, I felt I had indeed had, in another way, *a stroke of genius*!

Chapter 2

Touched By An Angel

In late October 1993, about a month before my stroke, my friend Rose invited me to a black-tie, gala concert at Old School Square, Delray Beach's restored cultural center. She asked that I sit beside her at her table because she wanted me to meet her friend Jan, who sat next to me. Seated on the other side of Jan was Emily, another very attractive lady. As it turned out, that meeting would have a profound impact on my life. I am sure neither Jan nor I could have known what a significant bond of friendship would result from our meeting that happy night.

I had to leave the party early that evening because I had to rise very early the next morning to fly to Japan on behalf of The Morikami Museum and Japanese Gardens. I was to thank our significant contributors in Miyazu, Japan. After two weeks in Miyazu, I flew back home and contacted Jan.

I scheduled a dinner engagement with her for November 28th, eleven days after my return from Japan.

That very afternoon I suffered my stroke. I still remember calling her right after I called 911. "Jan, I'm sorry I won't be able to make dinner this evening. I think I've had a stroke." Those were the words I meant to say, and what I thought I said to Jan. She later told me she only heard garbling sounds, not one clear word, but, recognized my voice if not my words. She became concerned and called my brother Ernie and told him about my call saying, "I think something very bad has happened to Sandy. You'd better look into it. He just called me and I didn't understand a word he said." Roy was already on his way to my apartment and so was the emergency rescue team. After I was taken to the hospital, Roy contacted Ernie, my third brother Charlie, and Jan. Soon they were all at Bethesda Hospital on vigil as I was placed in the Intensive Care Unit. Recognizing the gravity of my situation, my rector, Rev. Bernie Pecaro, was also notified and present, in the event that last rites would be needed.

While I remember very little about the first three weeks, I do remember Jan visiting me nearly every day during the balance of my hospitalization, spending time by my bedside, talking with me, counseling, and praying. She was always so gentle, so caring, so loving, and quite beautiful. Jan became very important to me. I finally asked her why I had become so important to her.

Here is her response to my question and why I liken Jan to Monica who appears weekly on my television set in the series *Touched By An Angel*.

"My dear friend Emily, whom you met at the Old School Square gala, is a very spiritual, religious person as am I. By now, you know both of us are born-again Christians. Several weeks before you and I met at the gala, I had told Emily that I had had a dream, and in that dream, there was a man in a wheelchair. He

needed my help and I went to him. After I told Emily about your stroke, she told me, 'Jan, you must go to Sandy. He is the man in the wheelchair and it is your calling to go to him. You must convince him God loves him and that God has healed him. He does not fully believe it nor do his doctors or his family. It is your obligation to convince Sandy that God loves him and he will be healed. And he must believe. He must have faith, for he needs a miracle of God to live, to survive this terrible stroke. And he must believe it is so. You must convince him.'

Emily convinced me to go to you, and I too was convinced with all my heart, all my being, Sandy, that you had already been healed by God. And even though no one else seemed to believe it, I did, and I was sent to convince you.

When I went to the hospital, you were in the ICU and I wasn't allowed into your room. Only family members were permitted and they visited you, but I couldn't. Your brother Ernie came to me in the waiting room after speaking with the doctors who had looked at the CT scans and MRIs. The doctors gave you very little hope. They said you might not make it through the night. Your brothers were very sad. They felt helpless watching their youngest brother so close to death. Ernie put his hand on my shoulder, looked into my eyes with tears in his and told me, 'Jan, I'm sorry you didn't know Sandy well. You would have liked him. But now you will never have that opportunity.' I felt so sad for him and so I embraced your brother, hugged him, and together we cried. Then I said to Ernie, 'Let's pray. I believe God has already healed Sandy and we must pray together to thank Him.' And we did."

During the next three months, my new friend Jan came to visit me often. She spent a lot of time with me. She talked with me, prayed for me, and nurtured my emotional understanding. Her visits gave me hope. She was understanding, kind, and so very patient. During the first month, she told me, my eyes were usually closed. Even when I couldn't speak well and suffered those constant hiccups and headaches, Jan was there. I could hear her and I could understand what she was saying, but most of the time, I couldn't respond so she could understand me.

There were other visitors as well, loving friends, men and women. Some were from my high school days, like Patsy who inspired me by holding my right hand while saying, "Sandy Simon, you rascal! Get well! If you had asked me to marry you when we dated in high school, I would have said 'yes' and you would have been taken care of so well you never would have had this stroke."

They came to my bedside and visited with me, encouraged me and conveyed their friendship and their belief in me. But Jan's visits were *different*. They were part of her mission. She had to convince me to *believe!* Hers was not a mission of sympathy or even empathy. While compassionate, she was reaching into my soul to convince me that God loved me and had already healed me. She did so by extending her hand to me, embracing me, praying with me, and leading me.

And so, I came to look forward to Jan's visits and called her on the phone when I missed her terribly. I remember calling her one chilly day in late December when I was feeling really cold in my bed. My room was at the end of the corridor and, even after I alerted the nurses, the hospital couldn't make my room any warmer. At the time, I was without a roommate for about a week and felt very much alone too.

"Jan," I asked, "can you come to the hospital and help me? I am very cold. I need your help." It didn't take her long. Jan suddenly and wondrously appeared at my bedside.

"Hi, Sandy," she said as she smiled that wide, beautiful smile. "I brought you something."

She pulled a softly knitted white cotton afghan from her tote bag. It was perfect, and I still use it.

One night in early March, during my third month in the hospital, I remember I telephoned Jan at her home. I'm not sure what prompted me, but I'm glad I did. Before the conversation ended, Jan prayed for me and with me.

"Do you believe God loves you?" she asked me.

"Yes!" I replied.

"And will you believe that through Him God is healing you?" she continued.

"Yes!" I quickly responded again.

"Then pray with me, Sandy."

We did. That night I turned over my life to God and it made all the difference. I gave up control.

The next day, my minister, Rev. Bernie Pecaro, came to my bedside, as he had so many times. "Pray for me, Bernie," I asked. "Will you ask God to heal my left arm which has not moved in nearly three months?"

"Of course I will, Sandy." And he did. And I believed I was being healed. I felt a wonderful sensation in my body I had not felt before as he prayed. As I committed and believed, I felt, with great emotion, that God had touched me and my atrophied left side was actually being healed.

I came to feel that Jan, so full of goodness, beauty, tenderness and love, personified what a true angel sent by God must be, and how fortunate I was to have met her. But, I often wondered, how and why did our meeting happen at that gala just before my stroke? Recently, I asked Jan and we began a very lengthy and wonderful conversation. Jan's every thought, every belief is of God which comes from her deep spirituality.

"There are no coincidences, Sandy. We were meant to meet. Consider this," she continued, "I had not attended a formal gala without a date in years. I just never would. The only reason I attended the Old School Square gala was because my friend Emily was visiting me for the weekend and she said she would go. If she had balked for any reason, I would not have gone. And, Sandy, don't forget, you would normally have taken a date but you had recently had a change in a personal relationship. Certainly it was not your style to go to a black-tie affair without a companion. If you had, we would likely not have met that night. I truly believe that God intended for us to meet at that time. God chose a time when we would be at our best and just about as charming as we could be."

Even today, nearly seven years later, I am convinced that Jan was sent to me as an instrument of God's love to help look at myself, my world, and my new place in it. She came to me in human form, full of grace and the Holy Spirit to show me God's unconditional love.

"Anyone in as much difficulty and pain as you were, Sandy, needed someone to look forward to seeing all the time and someone who would be there for you. You needed a person who *believed* you were going to get well, that you would be okay and that God had already healed you. Despite the doctors' visions, their views and opinions, the circumstances, your severe brain damage, your weakness, your pain, your paralysis you were in at that time," Jan spoke so softly, but confidently, "God wanted you to depend on Him, not only on yourself. He wanted you to believe deeply in His unconditional love for you, that He was aware of your condition and your pain, and that He wanted me to be with you to remove from you your doubt in Him and to come to Him. He knew your stroke was a result of your depending on yourself all your life. He allowed the stroke to happen and for you to live through this most severe and painful experience so that you would have the opportunity to turn from a religion *about* God to a relationship *with* God."

Jan had come into my life with a purpose. Her love of God, I truly believe, brought me from the depths of my lonely hell physically and emotionally to a place where I began to believe that I was loved and was not alone. Her beliefs and her visits inspired me to become more determined than ever to do everything I could to get well again.

I believe that angels are brought into our lives when we open ourselves to them, need God's guidance, and have absolute faith. They teach us to look at ourselves, our world, and our place in it. They can show us a new way of life with meaning we never saw before. I believe this is why Jan came into my life. Jan's message convinced me that with God's help, and my complete faith and determination, I would survive this ordeal.

Chapter 3

The Therapeutic Experience

Starting Over

Finding happiness after any personal catastrophe is a difficult mission to be sure. Whatever it is, a stroke, loss of a loved one, (especially the loss of a child), divorce, or financial disaster, it requires enormous strength, courage, determination and a positive perception of life. A great sense of humor was, in my case, essential. I was forced to come face to face with the harsh realities of the impacts of my severe stroke. I had lost my health. I was trapped in a body that wouldn't work. I surely could not do the things I used to do. I couldn't sit without falling over, I couldn't stand, I couldn't see to my left, and my entire left side was numb. Because my left arm was essentially flaccid, I couldn't even propel myself in a wheelchair. I was physically powerless and my personality changed radically. Where I had been an accomplished, confident, optimistic businessman and civic activist, I realized that I could *not do* those things I needed to do to accomplish the simplest tasks. That was my new life.

I was angry about it. I was deeply depressed. Thinking like that and having that negative perception is self-defeating. I desperately wanted to get back to my life before the stroke. But I couldn't. For months I fought the physical and emotional reality. It was the most demanding struggle of my life. And it continues, though I have improved greatly.

Physical therapy is normally begun within two or three days after a stroke. In my case, because my stroke was so severe, I wasn't sent to Pinecrest Rehabilitation Hospital for about five days. On my first day at Pinecrest, a "transporter" (a volunteer person) strapped me in a wheelchair and wheeled me to the elevator, then down one floor to the therapy gym. It was a large room, probably 50 feet by 80 feet, with large padded but firm mats on legs about two feet above the floor.

Rebecca, my physical therapist, recently recalled our first meeting — my behavior and my condition — that first day. Here are her words:

"As you were wheeled into the gym by one of the transporters, this is what I saw. You were slumped down in the wheelchair (like in a recliner chair) leaning over to the left with your right arm draped over your head, and a lap posey belt around your waist for safety. Your eyes were closed. You had a hard time keeping your feet on the footrests. I immediately motioned to the transporter and we met over at the quiet treatment room. I wheeled you into this room that was dimly lit and peaceful, away from the light, noise and voices in the gym. I closed the door and sat down on the mat beside you while you were in the wheelchair. I waited silently for about five minutes and then I said, 'Hello.' You responded immediately, in a whisper, with 'Hello.' I introduced myself and asked you to take a look at me so you would recognize me in the future. You

opened your eyes about one-quarter of the way and smiled a half-smile and then immediately shut them again. I then asked your name and you replied, 'Sandy.' Then I asked, 'Do you know where you are and why you are here?' Your quiet reply was, 'Yeah, I'm here to learn how to improve my golf swing.' With that, you assumed the position of hitting a golf ball. You leaned forward, although you really leaned to your far left, stretched out your right arm and began to swing your arm across your body in a motion like you were on the golf course or driving range. Your eyes stayed closed.

Understanding your confusion, I slowly explained to you that you were actually in a hospital, that you had suffered a stroke and that I would be working as your physical therapist.

Your reply was, 'Really?' You wrinkled your forehead and then said, 'Huh?' with a questioning expression on your face.

I think you really weren't aware of your stroke at the moment and truly thought, somehow, you actually were trying to improve your golf swing. You began showing your hyper-stroke-induced impulsiveness. I watched you attempt to take the actions I was describing to you before I was finished explaining the action to you. You were highly impulsive and compulsive at the same time. I explained to you that it was okay to be confused. I then asked you if you would like to get out of the wheelchair and sit on the mat.

Your response was, 'Sure.'

Even with your eyes closed, you immediately attempted to get up from the wheelchair and the constraining posey belt reminded you that you could not stand unrestrained.

I said, 'Sandy, wait for just a moment while I undo the belt and wait for me to give you a hand.' Then

I asked you if you would open your eyes to see where the mat was located.

You looked over at the mat and then closed your eyes again.

After that, we worked together to transfer you over to the mat from the wheelchair and moved you to a sitting, balanced position. You fell over to the left, unable to balance yourself in a sitting position. We took several quiet time breaks so as not to over-stimulate you.

During one of the breaks you said, 'Boy, that fan is loud!' There was an air-conditioning vent right above our heads. This was an example that emphasized your acute awareness of noises.

I then had you lie down on your back and worked on helping you roll from side to side, and then I assisted you back into a sitting position. You still required minimal assistance, about 25% from me, to sit and total assistance, 100% from me to transfer you back into the wheelchair.

*Our assistant, your transporter, and I returned you to your room and left you sitting in the wheelchair. We were saying good-bye and you said, 'Hey, Rebecca, I've got a joke for you. What is the difference between a man who is bald in the front, bald in the back, and men who are bald from front to back? The men who are bald in the back are lovers, the men who are bald in the front are thinkers, and the men who are bald from front to back **think** they are lovers!' With that you started laughing out loud at your own joke. Your roommate started laughing and I started laughing. That's when I noticed that your head was bald from front to back and I started laughing all over again.*

It was a positive sign. You were able to recall a joke, process the joke, verbalize it to me, use your right arm for appropriate gestures as you rubbed the top of your head, and you really had a great punch line! I immediately felt confident that we would make great strides in your rehabilitation and that you were an excellent candidate for all therapies. However, the next day was a totally different story.

The following day, when the transporter brought you to the gym, I immediately knew you were not the same man I had met the day before. I wheeled you into the quiet treatment room. You appeared sedated in some way. I called the nurse and asked if your medications had been changed. She replied that they had not. (First alarm.) I spoke to you and your response was very slurred, much more than the day before. (Second alarm.) We transferred you to the mat and even your right leg wasn't helping during the transfer. (Third alarm.) In sitting, you were actually falling backward and requiring total assistance (100%) from me to sit compared to the day before when you had only needed minimal assistance (25%) from me.

It became clear to me at that point that your condition was deteriorating rapidly. I was convinced I had to take action right away. I felt if we delayed, we might lose you. I immediately told you I was going to put you back in the wheelchair and I didn't want you to help me. I strapped you in with the posey belt for your safety and took you back to your room. I alerted the nurse, your physician and your family as quickly as I could."

Looking back, I cannot recall any specifics of my first days in the therapy gym. I do remember speaking with Rebecca, and being strapped in that wheelchair. And I am told that within minutes after Rebecca returned me to my room and met with my doctors and brothers, preparations were made to race me back by ambulance to Bethesda Hospital's intensive care unit for more tests and treatment. That's where I stayed for nearly a week while they sought to relieve the pressure in my brain.

I remember, as I lay in my hospital bed the first awful month, my brother Charlie telling me as sympathetically and lovingly as he could, "Well, Sandy, you'll have to look at this as taking a year out of your life." That observation was very candid and honest. His statement was instantly depressing to me, and I was startled with his observation. However, it has lasted much, much longer than a single year. I remember replying to my dear brother, "A year! I can't lose a year! How can I do that?" My life before, so active, so *busy*, flashed before my eyes. I didn't want to lose that life that I knew so intimately. I began that part of the cycle of grief called "bargaining." I said, "Maybe three months — maybe six months — but not a YEAR!!!!" (I thought) I had too much *to do*! Looking back, I had no reasons for challenging his observation. I was reaching for some basis to limit the damage this stroke was doing to my life. I was still in my "keep busy" accomplishment-oriented "don't waste time and don't be frivolous with life — be active" syndrome.

Later that day while I was alone, I thought about my brother's statement. All of a sudden my impairments, my separation from my world had a verbalized time period. A year before I could resume my life?...A year before I could walk?...A year before I could be independent?...A year before I could be productive again?...A year...

As I thought about this new reality, I found this to be a specified and quantified shock to my view of life. Up to that point, all anyone would say at the hospital, if I asked when I would be able to go back to work, was, "We don't know...we don't know...all strokes are different." "Will I walk again?" "We don't know." "How long until I know?" "We don't know."

"When will my left arm move?" "We don't know. It may never move again." Now I heard from my brother whom I trusted, "Think about it as giving up a year of your life." One year... There were no promises given. No one said, as they might with a broken arm or leg or even a heart by-pass operation, "Six weeks and you'll be as good as new." Or even, "Mr. Simon, in one year you'll be walking again." No, I never had anyone tell me anything remotely close to that. And how I wished someone could have. How much I hoped someone, someday would say, "Mr. Simon, only six weeks to go and you'll be walking in the park." It never happened. There was no brass ring for me to grasp. There were no trophies, no stated accomplishments in a definitive time period and no real life ring to give me hope.

But still, I was able to find the determination to pursue the "therapeutic experience" and actually began to look forward to each of my therapy sessions. I prayed to God incessantly for strength, for hope, for help, for a miracle.

I had daily sessions in psychotherapy with Dr. Maureen Lynch who really helped me immeasurably in rebuilding my self-esteem, understanding what had happened to me, and finding a way to reach acceptance. This was a terrible emotional disaster. During those sessions, we dealt with emotional issues like the enormous degree of anger I felt. And guilt...for any and all behavior of my past relationships that didn't work. And fear...How will I relate to people? What businessperson will want to work with me? I'm 56 years old, single, and don't believe any woman will even look at me again, much less be interested in a relationship. What about my sex life? There is so much garbage that has to be expunged from one's life so that one can move on.

Kerry, my occupational therapist, came each morning to dress me and to teach me activities of basic living using my right hand only. She spent a great deal of time teaching me to put my glasses on over both ears. Since my left side was without feeling, I couldn't tell if the arm of my glasses was over, on or around my left ear. All I could tell was that sometimes everything became blurred. She worked on my left arm and shoulder to prevent severe muscle spasms and pain. She showed me how to wash my right hand and nails using a stiff brush with suction cups on the bottom since I couldn't, and still cannot, wash both hands with a bar of soap as in days gone by. I couldn't stand, so I had to be wheeled to the sink.

Samantha, my speech therapist, not only helped me regain my ability to speak, but worked with me so patiently to rid my face of "left side droop" and make it symmetrical again. She would instruct and require me to do many strenuous, but necessary repetitive facial and tongue exercises. I looked like Joe E. Brown moving my mouth around, but it sure helped. The same difficulties with the tongue and throat muscles affected my speech and my inability to swallow. I could not stick my tongue out straight. When I tried for Samantha, it would veer sharply to the left. I couldn't control the left side of my tongue just like I couldn't control my left arm or leg. The right side therefore overpowered the left side and my lips and tongue would swing to the left. I felt great embarrassment. The only way I could point my tongue straight out was to look into the mirror and focus with a lot of concentration pointing my tongue, as much as possible, straight-ahead. At first I couldn't do it. But Samantha persisted for weeks and weeks, instructing me and encouraging me to try. It was so depressing at first. After all, this simple thing of sticking out your tongue as any child can do seems so easy, but when you've had a brain injury it is very difficult to do. That is very discouraging. The simplest tasks magnified the difficulty and seemed to be as hard to do as climbing a rugged mountain without shoes. Samantha would count as I stuck my tongue out at myself 40 times before she would let me rest. After a few minutes, she would make me repeat the effort. We had to train my undamaged, adjacent brain cells to "do it right"! I had to repeat these mouth exercises as many times as I could in my room while looking in the mirror. It took a lot of concentration, focus and determination. Eventually it got easier. Today, I am happy to say, my face is symmetrical and my tongue is back under my control.

Rebecca, my physical therapist, did say to me, as the one person who delivered a life ring as thrown from a boat to a drowning person, "Stick with me and we'll get you there!" She was so convincing and so sure of herself that I took on her confidence. I found that I absolutely could not disappoint her or myself. So I pushed myself to follow her instructions. Daily, she exercised me, counseled me, encouraged me, and eventually taught me to sit without falling over — and even to stand for half a minute. I remember watching the clock the first time I stood up. Five seconds...ten seconds...thirty seconds! Wow! Thirty seconds without tipping over and falling down. A miracle! She has since reminded me that, in the beginning, I told her, "All I want to learn is how to get from my wheelchair to my desk at work." I am amazed today at my simplistic, yet work-oriented goals.

After six weeks of therapy, I could stand at an angle, like the Tower of Pisa, leaning to my strong right side, but I could not take a step by myself. I didn't know where my left side was even after twelve weeks of constant therapy. During hours and hours of her therapy, Rebecca taught me to transfer weight from one foot to the other, even though I had no idea where my left leg was! So how could I shift my weight to the left? How far would I shift? Taking a step would be a miracle if I could eventually do it. But Rebecca never gave up on me. Each morning as I began getting more positive and accepting, I would say to the mirror, "Another day of therapy, another step toward independence and freedom."

My therapists and their assistants were encouraging, nurturing, energetic, young, and hard working. I couldn't understand where they got their reserves of energy. How, day after day, they could empathize (not sympathize) with, instruct, encourage and support people who were like me and who needed them so desperately. Their total commitment to their patients seemed to have no limits. That propelled me to commit myself to do my best, my utmost. It was painful, difficult and, especially, exhausting. Sometimes I got very sad when I couldn't do something simple like hold a large plastic ball between my knees while lying on my back. I even cried at my inability to control my left leg muscles. "Don't cry, Sandy, that's a very hard thing to do at this stage," encouraged Rebecca.

I was always tired. Even so, I was the last patient to leave the therapy gym every day. I was determined to perform all the therapy tasks I could so that I could never look back and say, "What if I had done more?"

I gradually realized that helping others, if only with a smile, energized my therapists and other patients. I used my sense of humor all I could. I learned from them that through giving I could change the lives of others, and that one truly does receive more than one gives. I received new energy, a renewed sense of reliance on the resilience of the human spirit and other intangibles. I began to grow as a person as I interacted with these wonderful people and I felt a sense of healing taking place within me. Emotional and cultural healing exceeded my physical healing. God *was* healing me faster than I thought when I looked at my flaccid, unfeeling left arm. Still, I was often sad and depressed with the severe impact on my life by this stroke.

Each day five to six hours of therapy followed the day before. I had no idea how long I would be in the therapeutic hospital, I had no deadlines per se or expectations to deal with — just today. Tomorrow would come. Yesterday was too painful to think about (though I did think longingly about the yesterdays before my stroke). I began to evolve into a state of "today." I would coach myself each morning saying, "Today I will achieve this or that. I will be positive, I will be optimistic." I found that if I could respond positively to the friendliness of the therapists, assistants and other hospital personnel who were so supportive, friendly and encouraging, then my day would be brighter, happier and more optimistic. Perhaps my behavior would give them back a bit of what they were giving me.

One day when I was feeling as if my life was never going to get better than this life of daily therapy and inability to coordinate the muscles in my body, a man came to me in his wheelchair. I was in the gym sitting on the elevated mat doing my leg exercises. It was mid-January 1994, my second month at Pinecrest Rehabilitation Hospital. His nickname was Charlie O. Later I found out that his real name was Charles Otto. Charlie O had experienced a severe stroke and, because of complications, was not able to swallow or eat anything by mouth for a long time. A "G-Tube" had been placed directly into his stomach so that he could receive nourishment. At the time he visited with me, he was an outpatient and was still in his wheelchair; yet, he was very upbeat, cheery, and friendly.

Rebecca had told me that it would be good for me to speak with Charlie O — and she was so right. Charlie O had sustained one of the worst strokes Rebecca had ever seen. I might have reached his condition had my bleeding not halted when it did.

Charlie O told me as we sat facing each other that he thought he was going to die only a few weeks earlier. He couldn't eat or swallow at that time, but he had progressed amazingly to his current place. He was in the preliminary stages of learning to stand and walk. He had a great positive attitude.

Charlie O's energy, passion and optimistic attitude were so infectious. I listened to his every word as he told me what he had been through. In many ways it was similar to my experience and in some ways worse than I had endured. Having someone come to you who has "been there" i.e., a "veteran" or a "native" as the therapists refer to people like Charlie O, is a major emotional experience and meant to be of significant inspiration in one's recovery. In my case, it was very empowering. Charlie O's visit to me was what I needed at the time. I think I was at a crossroads. I remember thinking this is too great a burden for me, that maybe I can't endure this recovery! Then, after his visit, my attitude began to change. I recall thinking, if Charlie O can do it, I can do it! Finally, I had met someone who had beaten the odds. I needed this messenger.

His visit did its work. I became enthusiastic and upbeat. I began believing that I *could* get better, significantly improve my station in life and look toward the future with a new sense of confidence and optimism. I felt I could "do like Charlie O did." From that moment on, I determined, with conviction, that I *would* walk again…that I would help and counsel other stroke victims and do all I could to empower other people who have suffered a stroke. The gift I received from Charlie O would be my gift to other stroke survivors. Charlie O was 76 years old at the time we visited and today, seven years later, Charlie O continues his current therapy three times each week. He's walking now, so most of his therapy is directed at bringing back his arm and hand. Charlie O recently said to me, "I'll just keep on with my therapy, improving little by little." He continues his therapeutic experience, as must we all.

One night, while lying in bed, I was thinking that I had to find the inspiration to sustain the determination to overcome my seemingly insurmountable challenges. I remembered that awful night in 1958 when I was in my junior year at Georgia Tech's School of Architecture. I had called home to tell my family I wanted to leave school and go back home. I was in a terribly desperate state because that semester I had had so much bad luck. I was totally exhausted and felt defeated. The project that my class had been assigned was to be graded the next day as the equivalent of a mid-term exam. Like several others, I had spent weeks, and finally, four days and four nights continuously working on that deadly exercise unique to the School of Architecture, the charrette. A charrette is an intensive final design project due before a specified deadline, and to me it was giving everything you had until you virtually collapsed from exhaustion. I really think charrettes are meant to convince some students not to continue to pursue architecture as a career.

That night I was so discouraged because some teenage vandals had come into the lab while we were out for dinner and destroyed all our work and all our efforts only about 12 hours before the jury was to review our projects! I was depressed and ready to quit school. So, like several classmates, I called home.

After I explained to my father and mother, (who had worked hard for my future, financed my education, suffered through the Great Depression, the years of World War II and other difficult times), that I wanted to leave school, my mother was, in her loving and understanding way, sympathetic. But my father said, "You've never quit before and you can't do it now. Don't come home if you quit. We have no room for quitters. Leave school if you choose, but don't come here."

Well, it was a difficult pill to swallow, but his "tough love" worked when I was 20 years old and the memory of that telephone conversation worked again 36 years later. Quitting now as a stroke survivor was not an option. I would not survive in a padded bed with Valium as my main diet.

So I resolved I had to find another way.

To be sure, there were many days and there were many nights when I was so depressed, so unhappy, so miserable. I couldn't move my body. My left leg felt like a dead log. My left arm was seemingly always in the way. Sometimes my left limbs would get caught in the bed rails but when that happened, I couldn't feel it and I didn't know I was in trouble.

Once, when my arm was caught and I couldn't turn, I called for the doctor. When he kindly came to my bedside, I told him, "I want you to cut off my left arm, here, at the shoulder." I pointed with my right hand. Irrational? Of course. But there are times of "giving up" that certainly are not all rational. He must have thought I had completely lost it. He gently responded, "We'll discuss it in the morning." I'm so glad one of us was thinking rationally.

And too, there were some very funny times. My bladder was really affected, and one time was simply out of control. It wasn't getting the right messages. When I was full I felt empty; when I was empty, I felt full. It was scary and weird. I was collecting and holding what seemed like quarts of urine for some unknown reason. It got so bad that I came close to "having a gusher" in my bed. Of course I didn't actually go to the bathroom; I used a portable, plastic bottle with a bent neck, and "expelled" (as the nurses called it) in the comfort of my bed. When I did, I virtually filled the bottle and it would spill over onto my bed. That was bad! It was comfortable until I didn't aim right. Then it was very uncomfortable and I was very wet! But holding the bottle and holding "Mr. Happy" at the same time with one hand was a juggling act, and I was never good at juggling!

So I called my doctor and said, "Please help me doctor, I'm full of urine." (I actually used the word "pee.")

Within a couple of hours, a nurse came to see me with an instrument they used to obtain a sonogram. It's the gadget they rub on an expectant mother's belly to see if the baby is going to be a boy or girl. Well, you can imagine how confused I was. I was thinking I had to go to the bathroom when I didn't, and thinking I didn't when I did. And now it seemed they were checking on a baby in my belly! The first thing the nurse did was smile and rub thick cool jelly on my stomach. Then she placed this heavy cylinder-like gadget on the electric transmitting jelly and rubbed it on my stomach while together we looked at a scope somewhat like those depth scopes they use on fishing boats to locate schools of fish or reefs. As she rubbed the sono-gadget on my stomach over my bladder, I looked at the screen with her. I said, "It looks like a school of fish there — let's drop 'the hooks'," (fishing jargon I thought she'd find funny). She didn't.

Well, after she left with her results, my muscular male nurse came to my bedside with his so familiar smile. "What's happening?" I asked him. "You're going to have a urine stress test," was his response.

He lifted me out of the bed and into my wheelchair and strapped me in. (God, I hated that strap!) Down the corridor we went to a small room occupied by a very capable, very muscular and very large woman dressed in white hospital slacks and blouse.

I didn't know what to expect, but judging from the imposing size of the nurse in the room and my helpless condition, I knew it would be futile to resist anything she wanted to do to me. "Upsy-daisy *ve* go," she smiled as she lifted me onto the bench from the wheelchair. (She said *ve* not *we*, so I called her Helga, the Swedish wrestler.) Well, it wasn't exactly a bench. It was one of those elevated padded tables doctors have in their offices.

As I sat on this bench or table with my legs draped over the side, Helga reached to the opposite table and picked up a long flexible tube that looked like a giant Dixie straw you get at a fast food restaurant. It was about three feet long and slightly larger in diameter than a drinking straw. As I stared at this "pipe," mentally comparing it to the size of my pitiful penis (after about two and a half months of solitary hospitalization), I couldn't believe she was going to do what I began to realize she *was* going to do. I watched her carefully and asked the stupid question, "What do you think you're going to do with **THAT**?"

Then, after she described how she was going to catheterize me, I said, "Not with that fire hose you're not, it's bigger that I am!"

Then she said, "Close...your...eyes...!"

"Ulp!"

"Now," she said, "*ve* are going to fill you up with saline water. Tell me *vhen* you feel you are full."

I gasped, "Are we talking a pint? Gallons?" I began to perspire. "That looks like a five gallon bottle. Have you ever done this before?" I couldn't stop talking. "They call this nervousness...I'm full! What is that?"

"I'm going to remove this Dixie straw, er...catheter...and insert this new *von*."

I yelped, " But it's even bigger." I tried to convince her to stop. No luck.

"It's in now and *ve* are going to empty you. Tell me when you think you are empty."

When she was done with that task, I watched Helga reach to the shelf and grab a spool of wires about ten feet long.

"What are you going to do with those?" I begged.

"*Ve*" (she kept saying 'we' like I was helping her) "are going to attach these wires to your scrotum and then to the speakers on the shelf."

"What? Do you think you're going to broadcast my groin saying 'hubba-hubba' as I watch the pretty nurses walk by the door? Are you a sicko?"

This whole episode was embarrassing and frightening...and seemed ridiculous to me. "What am I going to do about this 'problem' when I'm out of the hospital?" I asked Helga, who did not respond. Still there was something about it that was sickeningly funny. "Does your mother know what you do for a living?" I teased her. And thankfully she laughed.

During my residence at Pinecrest in January and February 1994, the announcements of the 1996 Atlanta Olympics were in all the media. I really wanted to go to the Olympics! I had long wanted to attend the Olympics at least once, and now they were being held in Atlanta, my favorite city where I had many friends. I love Atlanta, and the idea that the Olympic Village would be on the campus of Georgia Tech triggered all sorts of nostalgia and great collegiate memories for me.

But reality slapped me in the face. "You will have great difficulty trying to go to the Olympics," I was told. "Hardly anyone can get tickets. You'll be in a wheelchair. You can't even *think* of the Olympics. They're so spread out. It is out of the question. You're dreaming, Sandy. You can't go to the Olympics. You've suffered a massive stroke!" The admonishments went on and on.

But I felt the Olympics were too significant a goal for me not to seek. The idea of getting to the Olympics in June 1996, two and a half years hence, would give me a wonderful and powerful incentive to overcome my impairments and a timetable I could not extend.

So, I began two almost impossible tasks. The first was to focus on my grueling therapy and the second was to attempt an almost equally near-impossible requirement — I had to somehow figure out the maze of ticket application forms. (Remember how complex they were? All the newspapers and television programs commented one would need a computer to fill out the forms accurately.) They were quite a frustrating puzzle to me! Remember, I couldn't see to the left. In fact, though I sent them in after being convinced they were correct, together with payment, it turned out they were incorrectly done and were returned. I had to do them all over again. They were returned again. What to do? Call on NASA to help me? I sent them a third time. Success!

What was interesting was that my visitors, still questioning my sanity, would look at me with a dubious smile and comment, "Do you really expect to get tickets? And if you do, who is going to take care of you? You know you really can't expect to travel to Atlanta and attend the Olympics."

My response always was, with a smile, "I'm not ordering tickets, I'm applying for 'Javelin Catcher'!"

The experience of physical therapy remained my major focus, as I believe it is for most stroke survivors. Learning to walk again meant I could get around without always calling for help. It meant a degree of freedom. And it would be a major step in rebuilding my self-confidence. Working in the gym, two sessions each day, was a rigorous and painful experience. It was a humbling, sometimes bumbling way of life. I kept reminding myself that it was a necessary experience, and that through it, I was on my road to independence. So I did everything asked of me. If I had to do 20 "somethings," I did 25. For days, I stared at the training steps in the corner — four unpainted wooden steps with handrails. When I would ask why other patients were training on them and not me, Rebecca's answer, with great understanding and patience, would be, "Soon, Sandy, soon. Stay with the program, do what I ask, stick with me and you'll do fine on the steps. Their strokes weren't as severe as yours." So the steps became my goal.

In time, she took me outside to learn how to walk on the soft grass, then on gravel across a small inclined bridge. So simple before. So difficult now — but always getting easier. I really had trouble keeping my balance on soft or sloped surfaces, and my left ankle turned under all the time. Each step became a victory. Each new walking surface a new day, a new challenge. These inclines up and down...so difficult, so unsteady, so unbalanced. We would toss a beach ball to work on my sense of balance. Walking on gravel and soft grass was very difficult. Even today, I have difficulty with soft grass or thick carpeting. I was like a child learning to walk for the first time. But we adults fall farther and harder when we fall, don't we?

To rebuild my abilities, capabilities, confidence, self-esteem and my dignity, and achieving almost anything, became my entire focus. It's like building a giant earth dam, one stone at a time. And if you stay with it, don't give up — each achievement does become a victory. Figuratively, your mental shelves become full of trophies. My therapists were not only teachers and instructors; they were becoming my cheerleaders, my friends. Every victory was considered more reason for hope. Everyone in the hospital was "on my side." It became as though the universe was coming to help me, to encourage me, to applaud my every accomplishment. God's love? God's presence?

Sometime in late February, Rebecca and Kerry came together to my room to visit me. "Would you be willing to be our 'patient' as we perform a demonstration in front of the other therapists here at Pinecrest?" they asked me.

"What do I have to do? I can't do much, you know," I replied.

"We'll explain to the group of therapists the various positions a stroke survivor should be placed in while lying on the bed in order to protect the body, the limbs, and still ensure the comfort of the patient. It will take about 10-15 minutes."

"OK," I said, "I'll do whatever you want me to do."

"Also, we've heard you have given speeches before your stroke. Would you be willing to speak to the hospital's therapists and assistants and convey to them what it is like to be a stroke patient? We have to read and listen to lectures in our training, but always from the view of doctors, therapists, or hospital administrators. Rarely, if ever, do we hear what it's like from the patient's point of view. It would really be a wonderful thing for all of us if you would agree."

Well, Rebecca, Maureen, and Kerry were unselfishly giving me my life back, and for weeks I was the beneficiary of their devotion to my welfare and me. How could I possibly say no to their request? Besides, they knew, if I could succeed in this effort in front of over 70 therapists and assistants, it would be a major step in regaining my self-confidence and removing some of that emotional detachment we stroke survivors have to face.

As stated on the National Stroke Association web site, "The ability to define the world and our place in it distinguishes our humanity. Stroke forever alters this 'world-making capacity.' The stroke patient's world, once comprehensible and manageable, is transformed into a confusing, intimidating and hostile environment. The skills of intellect, sensation, perception and movement which are honed over the course of a lifetime and which so characterize our humanity are the very abilities most compromised by stroke. Stroke can rob people of the most basic methods of interacting with the world."

Sadly, I must concur with this observation. That is where I was as a stroke patient...disoriented and stiff, detached from others. Even today, when I watch the video taken of my 45-minute talk to the therapists at Pinecrest, I am reminded that I was experiencing these conditions. My voice was monotonous, without passion or enthusiasm. I seemed very stiff and unsure.

As I spoke standing at a podium, just a few steps from my wheelchair, I recall feeling confused, detached and intimidated even though I was an experienced speaker. The stroke had taken its toll in yet another way. In addition, for the entire time I spoke, Rebecca knelt behind me, massaging and slapping my legs so I would stand straight. My tendency was to put most of my weight on my right leg and hardly any on my left leg. It would take many months, even several years, before I would be able to discern standing vertically, not on a 5-10 degree list.

The opportunity to speak to this devoted and sympathetic audience was immensely beneficial to me and, I am told, also beneficial to the therapists. I am grateful to them for that experience. This was another major achievement that helped me regain a sense of self-esteem, "connection with others," and confidence, which were totally removed from me as a result of the stroke. I was totally humbled. I had no sense of self-worth, no confidence whatever, and, as Kerry, Maureen, Rebecca and all the other therapists must have felt, I am sure, that this speech would be a monumental step for me to re-establish a place in my world. I am told I rarely looked at those in the audience to my left, even though I tried to compensate by deliberately turning my body to my left. Not enough, as it turned out, but it was a beginning, and enabled me to have a sympathetic experience in interacting with the world. I would encourage this sort of experience in therapeutic hospitals. Effort should be made to program interactive experiences for survivors, even if only in small groups.

Seven years later, I understand that the video of my speech is still shown each year to the staff of rehab therapists who treat stroke survivors, and continues to be helpful to them. Speaking before this large group was especially significant for me.

Each morning at Pinecrest, I had breakfast with two kind ladies, both therapy patients. After we finished breakfast, I would always ask them if they would like me to read to them. Both would smile and say "yes." For one hour, I would read from a book of daily prayers and messages of hope entitled *God Calling*. Months later, when we met at the hospital by chance, we laughed together as they told me, "We listened as you read and most of the time we couldn't understand you. But we listened just the same and loved you for wanting to share with us. You were so happy to read." Due to my left side blindness, I did not see the first few words on the left margin of the next line. So, I always skipped several words! I slurred my speech too. No one corrected me. And no one understood me.

Biofeedback was a new therapeutic treatment available at Pinecrest, not universally approved by Medicare or insurance companies at the time. I learned of it in February 1994. I was in my third month at Pinecrest Hospital. My left arm had not moved one millimeter in three months and I had to do something, even if it was not covered or approved by my insurance company. "If your arm has not moved in three months, it probably never will." That was the message given me as I began seeking a biofeedback therapist. I would grasp any possibility of restoring my health and getting my left side to move…even a little.

Biofeedback was a new word to me and I had no idea what it was, how it worked, who did it or whether it was effective. All I knew about biofeedback was that more than two fellow patients had suggested I "look into it." So I did. I was eager to pursue *any* treatment that would help improve my condition.

I wanted to find this one person, Jim, a male therapist who not only was a biofeedback therapist, but was also a counselor on sex issues. The fact is, like most stroke survivors, I had no idea of the potential impact of stroke on my sex drive, my physical capabilities and how having sexual intercourse might affect my blood pressure. I had a lot of fear about this issue. I wanted to ask Jim some common questions, such as, Can I even think about having sexual intercourse again? Is that gone too? After all, I am only 56. If I do have intimacy, will I die in the act from another burst blood vessel in my brain? How do I manipulate my body when half of my body is beyond my power and feels like someone has given me a giant shot — actually, an overdose — of novocaine on my entire left side?

Jim was a very pleasant, helpful fellow and he was on the cutting edge of stroke *and* sex therapy, and biofeedback treatment in this new age of the boomer generation. I sought every bit of assistance available, including discussions with Jim. Of course, each visit had to be pre-approved by my insurance company and there was a limit to the number of visits. But even if my insurance didn't pay for it, I would have. The subject of sex was, well, pretty important to me. I think that is true of most adults. *Sex* is America's most obsessive subject and, I think it is safe to say, America's male preoccupation. I had to ask for guidance on this subject because it was not offered. But it is a very important issue that should be confronted.

I initially focused on the biofeedback treatments, especially on my left arm, which after five months, was immobile, flaccid and flopping around as if it was attached to my shoulder by a string. It was usually in the way. It was also a constant visual reminder of the impact of my stroke.

When I first visited Jim for biofeedback treatment in his small office cubicle, I saw what appeared to be three small television sets, which were actually monitors, on his table hooked to some sort of computer by a series of wires with electrodes of some sort. After explaining this (then) "new technique," Jim attached the electrodes to my left arm: two on my outer muscles, my extensors, and two to my inner forearm muscles, my flexors. After everything, including me, was hooked up, I was instructed to focus on the horizontal lines moving across the monitor screen left to right. The blue line represented my forearm outer muscles (extensors); the yellow represented the inner forearm muscles (flexors). I stared at the lines and at my left hand, trying as hard as I could to make something move...*anything*...my arm, my thumb, the blue line, the yellow line...*anything*.

After about ten minutes, Jim told me to stop. I was straining so hard, so determined and so focused, that I was dripping wet and yet nothing had moved. "Let's rest for a few minutes," Jim suggested. After a few minutes, we tried again...still, nothing moved. I was struck by the fact that after so much effort, and trying so hard mentally to consciously make a muscle or muscle group move even the slightest bit, nothing happened. Jim sensed my deep concern and sense of futility.

He told me, "Sandy, sometimes it takes several sessions. So let's go on to your questions regarding your future as it relates to sexual intimacy. Here are some drawings I think you'll find helpful. They depict relative positions you and your partner will find comfortable in view of your left side numbness and difficulty in moving." There were graphic depictions of a man and a woman partnering. Yippee! I thought — sex could still be in my future. For a few minutes, I forgot my sense of frustration and futility at the biofeedback monitors and thought about sexual intimacy.

"Jim," I asked softly, almost in a whisper, and with a bit of embarrassment and great reluctance, "are you saying to me, in the event I can find someone who one day may be interested in having intimacy with me, that I can physically do it, I can be able to please my partner, and I won't kill myself while I'm at it." (Although, I added to myself, if I've gotta go, that's the way to go!...will that make her a murderess?)

He laughed, "That's exactly what I'm saying, my friend. You can look forward to a full life. Don't give up. It's up to you."

I enjoyed his sense of humor and found great relief after our conversation. A major load of fear and apprehension had been lifted from my shoulders, so to speak. Not that sex was such a critical priority for me at that particular moment, but it was certainly on my mind a lot. Like everyday. Walking and using my left arm were also priorities, and so was speaking correctly. But being assured by Jim helped to give me a sense that I could become a complete and capable man again. And I have found that although initially I had numbness on the left side of *all* my body parts, in time, that numbness of a man's penis gradually goes away, especially, as with playing the piano, with lots of practice. Today, I am happy to say that everything works just fine, in fact better than ever! I am convinced of this because my lady friend doesn't smile just on her left side any more. (For progress reports, e-mail @ strokerehabstudguy.net or stroke rehabstudguyladyfriend.com.) Sometimes, it's only in the believing you *can* do something that helps rebuild one's self-esteem, dignity and sense of confidence. That's what I felt that day... "Another small step for mankind and one man's ego."

The following week, I met again with Jim in his office. He connected me up again with the biofeedback computer program that he said was created at the Miami Project, a terrific spinal cord research center at The University of Miami.

This time, I was determined something would move. After the contacts had been applied to my forearm muscles as before, and the monitor showed the blue and yellow lines, I began my effort once again.

"Concentrate on the lines," Jim instructed me, "Make them move."

I focused. I concentrated. I was determined. Five minutes...nothing.

"Rest. Try again," he said.

Ten minutes...nothing.

"Rest. Try again. Focus, Sandy, focus."

Harder and harder I tried. Perspiration began running off my forehead into my eyes. But nothing moved.

"Try to touch your left index finger to your thumb, Sandy. Try to make it move...tell your thumb to touch your index finger. Focus, Sandy. Get mad, Sandy. Order it to touch your forefinger. Say it out loud, Sandy. Make a circle with your thumb and forefinger, Sandy."

Fifteen minutes had passed. I was almost totally exhausted. I was dripping wet. I was amazed so much effort had gone into this simple thing that any child can do. Touch my thumb to my forefinger? So easy, I thought. Dammit. Push the throttle all the way, like getting the airline jet to move in the snow. Go for it. Give it everything you've got!

I reached deep inside and found strength they say can happen in critical situations. Perhaps, when a small person, a mother, saves her child by lifting a car weighing thousands of pounds. Somewhere, one can somehow tap into a source of strength, emotional and physical we didn't know we had.

As I found this strength, absolutely determined...stubborn?...and not willing to give up...I literally commanded my thumb to reach for my index fingertip and my index finger to bend toward my thumb. "Now!" I said aloud. "Do it!"

I watched with Jim as the blue line moved, so slightly, so did the yellow line. Then, I looked, and then stared at my left thumb and index finger. They moved! Slowly, ever so slightly toward each other. As they got closer to each other, moving maybe one-half inch each toward each other, I could feel my mouth twitch. Even my left foot moved.

Not there yet...I kept forcing myself. Go! Close the loop! Finally, I was exhausted. My thumb and forefinger *had* moved toward each other. They *had* closed the gap. They *had* responded, *finally*. And although they did not touch, they *had moved*! It was a beginning!

Yes. I had achieved a monumental accomplishment. My left hand had finally, after five long months, responded to a command.

Within a few days, I worked on my left foot with Jim, who once again connected my muscles to the computer with electrodes. After a lot of effort, I was able to move my left big toe. I was making progress! Enormous progress! Small accomplishments for sure, but one step at a time had become my daily goal.

Intensive therapy is one of the major means of returning one's body and mind to soundness. It takes total commitment of the stroke survivor to endure every session. It is exhausting, hard and painful work. There are no promises extended and no guarantees. But it can work in almost all cases.

The capabilities available to improve the quality of our lives has grown significantly over the past few years, become more effective, and yielded greater results than ever before due to ongoing cerebral/therapeutic research. The stroke survivor has good reason to look to the therapeutic experience for hope, progress, and eventual restoration. Caregivers must be lovingly firm and endlessly patient to keep the survivor focused and committed. Believe me, it's well worth the effort. "No pain, no gain" as they say. Stay with the program and you'll get there.

The therapies I experienced in the hospital made a major difference in my life. It continues even now, after all these years, and will likely continue for many more years, until I can use my limbs and walk without being in constant pain or exhausted.

Chapter 4

Coming Home

What to expect as an outpatient

On March 9, 1994, the 90th day after I was admitted to Pinecrest Rehabilitation Hospital, I was released. When I received my two weeks notice of discharge I was surprised because, physically, I still wasn't able to do much for myself. I was hoping I would be more independent before I had to be on my own. Also, emotionally, I didn't want to leave the hospital, my "warm, fuzzy home." I had grown attached to the hospital staff, my therapists and their total care. I felt secure and safe there.

And had to say good-bye to Rebecca. It was a wrenching, sad occasion for me. I owed so much to Rebecca, Kerry, and all the other therapists. Rebecca was an "inpatient therapist," and other "outpatient therapists," would now treat me. It wasn't the same, and I believe there is a sense of leaving the "warm womb" for patients when they leave the hospital for the "cold, cruel world out there." The thought of leaving the hospital made me feel apprehensive and uncertain about my unknown future.

All of those emotions were also accompanied with a sense of personal progress because I was about to enter a new phase in my life. I think everybody has them as they leave a hospital, a place where you feel you were well taken care of, where people nurtured you and where, indeed, your quality of life was dramatically improved. Yet, I knew I had a long way to go. Certainly there were mixed emotions. However, I did want to go home and resume my life in my "new" world.

The hospital required that I should be assisted out its doors in a wheelchair, for liability insurance purposes I suppose. I had sworn earlier that "my genes (weak blood vessels) may have gotten me into the hospital, but my genes (tenacity, determination and resilience) were darned well going to get me out." I was determined that I would "walk" out of the hospital, and in a manner of speaking, I did. The moment we passed the sliding hospital doors, I asked to be let out of the wheelchair so that I could walk the 20 feet to the curb and enter the car. I was wearing a fiberglass brace that fit around my left calf, around my ankle, and under my foot. Rebecca had placed this brace on my leg to give me extra security and to prevent "toe drop" that caused me to stumble. I could then focus on my trunk muscles and hips. I also walked with a cane in my right hand. I stood straight as a rod; so proud, so determined. I felt an enormous sense of accomplishment and pride having come so far from such a near hopeless place when I entered that hospital three months earlier.

I also felt good leaving some of the hospital life behind. How could I forget that dreadful three-wheeled little cart? The one with the wobbly, noisy wheel the morning nurse would push down the corridor to my bed at 4:30 a.m. After waking me to take my pulse and my blood pressure, she would give me a pill. What *was* that pill? Was it really a sleeping pill? Sometimes I thought, as I heard that wheel wobble toward my room for 100 feet, making such an obnoxious noise so early, please Lord, don't let that thing be coming to my bed. How I hated that noise. Do they deliberately make one wheel squeak? Eventually I assumed that all those carts were built with one bad wheel just to bother the hospital patients who were soundly sleeping — something like the Marine drill sergeant at boot camp, I suppose!

And how could I forget the food? I knew I would not miss the notorious hospital food so carefully cooked that no matter what choice you made the day before on the questionnaire, it always tasted the same, like unseasoned cardboard: no salt, no cholesterol, no fat, no taste. The only thing that I remember enjoying was the baked ziti. It wasn't pretty, but it did have flavor.

As I was about to get into the car to leave Pinecrest, Rebecca instructed me to back in carefully, sit down and then swing in my hips. Ena, my new aide, drove me to my apartment building about five miles away and wheel-chaired me from the car into my building. It felt strange somehow, being pushed through the lobby to the elevator and saying, "Hello" to neighbors for the first time in three months from a wheelchair. The last time they may have seen me was when I was wheeled unconscious on a rolling stretcher out the same front doors into a waiting ambulance. But *my* memories were of being healthy and "normal" while walking through that lobby.

My emotions were high, and I recall feeling a combination of excitement and happiness, but also lowered self-confidence, separateness and even needless embarrassment as a result of returning home in a wheelchair. It was a stark realization that having to turn my daily fate over to others was not limited to the hospital. It made quite an impact on my emotions. I felt sadness, yet I felt friendliness and sympathy from my neighbors. I wanted to cry. I was so sensitive. I cried at the drop of a hat. I was very vulnerable, like many stroke survivors.

And so, here I was, back in my apartment, home at last. I noticed some details that were different. Rebecca and Kerry had told me that they were going to inspect my apartment for safety corrections. I had an Oriental rug on the wall-to-wall carpet, but because together they were too soft for my walking ability, the rug had been put in storage. They were also afraid my left foot would catch the fringed edges of the Oriental rug, causing me to stumble. Chairs and a coffee table had been put into storage to remove obstacles in my path and give me more space.

In the bathroom, an elevated seat over the toilet was installed so that I could stand up by myself, using my atrophied thigh muscles. They had installed metal grab bars in the shower stall and a European-style hand-held showerhead with a flexible pipe so I could rinse my body using my right hand. A plastic chair was also placed in the stall because I could not stand for too long a period of time without losing my balance or getting tired. Stepping high while maintaining balance was not yet possible, so getting in and out of a bathtub to shower was totally out of the question. It wouldn't be possible for at least two years. Though I can now shower in a bathtub, I still can't lie down in the tub because I can't get up. For me, it would be like getting into a tub coated with olive oil. I'd probably die there unless someone rescued me! A Jacuzzi is still not a possibility.

But I was home! After looking around, I immediately went to bed. I was tired. And I would learn quickly that I would be tired much of the time. I napped after breakfast and I napped after lunch. I would have dinner at 5:30 p.m. and be in bed by 7 p.m. I played soothing music all the time on my tape/CD player. My favorite was the sound track of *Forrest Gump* — I really enjoyed the movie and the music.

For a few weeks, I had outpatient therapists come to my home until there was a place for me back at Pinecrest as an outpatient. The outpatient therapists didn't seem to be as effective or endearing as Rebecca and Kerry, but therapist assignments were in someone else's hands, not mine. I requested being treated by Rebecca because I knew I would progress faster and better with Rebecca. But the hospital was firm that Rebecca was an "inpatient therapist" only. I really missed Rebecca's instructions. In fact, I regressed in my ability to walk.

As I transitioned from hospital to home, my personality began to noticcably change. I became more and more docile, accommodating, and patient with the world. I was forced to accept the reality of my life. I couldn't do very much for myself or for anyone else. I began taking small doses of medication each day that helped my depression and anxiety.

Now that I had left the hospital with all its organization, nurses, aides, doctors, and multitudes of visitors, I regained a lot of the privacy that I had lost. I could awaken when I wanted for the first time in three months. I could visit my own bathroom, sit while I ate in my favorite chair, enjoy the view from my terrace and resume a semblance of my life before the stroke.

When I couldn't come to the phone at home after I left the hospital, I taped a message on my answering machine: "I'm sorry I can't come to the phone right now. I'm practicing the 'macarena,' and if I rush, I break furniture." This was, of course, in 1995 when President Clinton used the "macarena" song and dance as part of his campaign and it became a national favorite. It was my way of easing the caller with a bit of humor.

Other difficulties I had, most of which are milder now or not a serious issue any longer, included errors in judgement. My behavior, true to a right-brain injury stroke, caused me to have an exaggerated impulsive behavioral style. Sometimes, I thought I could do anything, (though I've not yet believed I can fly from my high-rise apartment balcony). For example:

The very night I left the hospital and went home, Ena, my maid, drove me from my apartment downtown to The Cornell Museum reception and fundraising event, taking my wheelchair in the trunk of her car. Then, after removing the wheelchair at the museum and getting me out of the car into the wheelchair, for the first time of my life I was wheeled up the ramp of a public building where many of my friends would see me post-stroke for the first time. I was nervous, probably feeling a lot of needless embarrassment and trepidation.

The event was wonderful. I was feted because of my recovery and because before my stroke I had helped arrange this successful opening, and the presence of well-known Jamaican artist, Guy Harvey, who was famous for his sea-life paintings that featured various species of fish. His works include, as examples, *The Dolphins* for the Miami Dolphins (the NFL team), *The Marlins* for the Miami Marlins baseball team and thousands of T-shirts featuring his fish paintings. Photos were taken all around. He and I were honored, very nice words were said, and I was wonderfully received. A lovely lady I had never met came over and introduced herself. She was so pretty and pleasant that I suddenly felt attractive — totally contrary to my post-stroke depression that robbed me of all self-esteem and sense of worth. Augusta couldn't have been nicer, lovelier or better for my self-confidence. She was in town for the winter season from Boston. Her timing couldn't have been more exquisite. And, of course, I was vulnerable to kindness. I felt no reluctance in imagining I was normal and not impaired...at least that evening.

Ena and I left the event at about nine o'clock and went back to the apartment. I couldn't take more than a couple hours in public my first night. Again, Ena loaded my wheelchair into the car, drove us home, removed the chair from the car, placed me in it, and parked the car. When she returned, she pushed me to the building door. En route, we bumped into the two-inch curb. Ena had to lean back my chair and push the front wheels onto the raised sidewalk. I found for the first time true empathy for those in wheelchairs powered by their own arms. I couldn't have overcome the curb by myself. It might as well have been four feet high...it was a huge barrier at two inches. This was another reminder of being life-impaired and wheelchair-bound. I fought off a sense of self-pity that crept up on me so often. Instead, I tried to hold onto who I was. Yet, I remember a great sense of being humbled. That's the sensation that I was feeling almost all the time: humility. I remember thinking God is teaching me a lot of lessons including humility.

We got to the apartment and I asked if Ena would take me to the bathroom. She did, and suggested I shower again as I'd had quite a workout.

Ena walked me to the bathroom, sat me on the smooth toilet seat cover and helped me undress. Thinking I was secure, she left me for a minute to go get another bath towel before walking me to the shower and setting me in the plastic chair there. My new way of taking a shower was sitting and using a hand-held showerhead on a flexible hose.

It was not a good idea for Ena to leave me alone. During that brief moment of separation, for some reason, I looked to my left, my blind side, and not having any feeling in my left "cheek," I confidently stretched and reached far to my left with my right hand, across my body, for a washcloth lying on the vanity top. I was a perfect example of the compulsive, impulsive behavior a right CVA injury stroke victim experiences. I *thought* I could reach so far to my left with my right arm. I *thought* I could tell with my right "cheek." I *thought* I was secure. But I wasn't. I started to fall off the toilet seat and got frightened about that. So, again my compulsive behavior took over and with my right hand, I did what the therapists told me *not* to do so many times, I reached for the edge of the hinged, movable door for support. As I grabbed the door, it moved as I moved and my hips hit the door as I fell. My body weight slammed the door against my fingers and squeezed them against the jam. The metal door lock was exactly where my fingers grabbed the edge of the door. As the door slammed, trying to fully shut, I pressed the door with my body weight and crushed my fingers in the door-jam space. I severely cut the index finger on my right hand, my only good hand and the one that I had already broken in the hospital six weeks earlier. The flesh was cut to the bone and I began bleeding profusely. I yelled for Ena who came running. Blood was everywhere and I was covered with blood. I was very frightened and mad at myself. I also felt sorry for myself and for Ena. Ena was frightened too and screaming at herself for leaving me. She kept repeating, "Dear Jesus, Lord Jesus, what have I done?" I felt like we were two children caught in an emergency beyond our capacity.

"Call the hospital. Tell them we're coming to the emergency room...get my clothes...wrap my finger...get me ready to go to the car...where's the wheelchair? Let's go quickly," I called out to Ena. She responded quickly to my needs.

Within fifteen long minutes, we reached the ER. My hand was still bleeding even with the bandage Ena had wrapped around my finger. After a while, a young doctor came to see me (they all seem so young now that I'm over 50 years old).

After two hours, cleansing of the wound, eleven stitches, and a lot of nervousness, Ena and I returned home very tired with two new, clear messages: Ena would not leave me alone again unless I was securely in bed, on the couch or in a large chair...nothing slippery, insecure or where I might be vulnerable; and I learned how dangerous and painful my new risky behavior could be unless I stopped myself. It was a rude awakening and a reminder of what my therapists had told me, that I had lost all common sense ability, at least for the first few months. What a night. It was after eleven o'clock when Ena finally put me to bed. We were both wiser and exhausted.

Disorientation is to be expected. All of these losses contribute to one's depression, especially when one never knows if these senses will ever return. Happily though, many of these problems began to dissipate during the first year.

I also had to swallow my sense of dignity and privacy at times. I was initially reluctant to have Ena, a woman I just met, see me naked as she bathed me while I sat on the plastic seat in my shower stall. She had to lather me, rinse me and dry me. I did reserve the right to do my own "privates." We both laughed when I said to her the first time, "Whoa, Ena, I get to do the 'good parts'."

Then again, she still had to pull down my pants or pajamas when nature called, wipe my bottom, then when finished, pull my pants back up. But, I soon began to feel relaxed with these experiences, having an unknown woman, very nurturing and considerate, see me naked and take care of my personal needs. Here comes that word acceptance again. And in a way, that is, metaphorically, coming home.

Ena was an excellent cook and companion. As a Jamaican immigrant, she always joked, "We Jamaicans make the best caretakers." I think I agree with her. Without any discussion, I could see I was "letting go" of control of my life, turning it over to God and to Ena, at least for the time being. I really needed a constant companion, friend, and someone who had no demands on me whatever. I grew very dependent on Ena as she took charge of my day-to-day life. We became friends. I was the patient, house-owner and, in a manner of speaking, the "bread-winner." But Ena, for the five months she stayed with me, had the run of my house, shopped, cooked, and kept me clean and comfortable. She even laughed with me at my jokes sometimes.

I was emotionally very fragile, vulnerable, and hypersensitive to just about everything — including friends, family, odors, and temperature changes. I had extreme senses of hearing, smell and taste. I found that cooking odors from the kitchen were very strong and obnoxious. I'd ask, "Ena, what's that awful smell?" Most foods tasted totally different from what I remembered. Sweets became too sweet and sours became too sour. I couldn't bear to eat some foods. I couldn't stand the sense of hyper-smell.

I would feel too cold or too warm without warning and call out, "Ena, please turn up the thermostat one degree." Even a one-degree temperature change was noticeable. I was also hypersensitive to sounds. "Ena, where is that loud noise coming from?" I had a bell by my bed (even that ringing sound was loud to me) to get Ena's attention at any hour so she could quickly respond to all my questions or help me to the bathroom, the shower or my chair for a meal. Can you imagine responding to such constant demands?

The first time I took a shower, it was a terrible experience. I felt the light water spray from the newly installed handheld water spray. It felt natural on my right side, but when the fine drops of spray struck the left side of my body, they felt like sharp knives piercing my skin. My brain was so confused and it misinterpreted the sensation so severely, that I screamed and cried from the severe pain. It was as if I was being stabbed like Janet Leigh in the terror movie *Psycho*. It was really terrifying and painful. I had to have Ena get me out of the shower quickly and put me in bed until the pain subsided. But today, that pain no longer exists...it gradually went away. "In time, all things pass" I am reminded. And many of these awful experiences over time do go away, thank God.

I am very grateful for Ena's inexhaustible patience and understanding. Today, I wonder how any caregiver, spouse, partner or family member would even be able to understand the apparently unreasonable and constant demands of a stroke survivor. There is a deep sadness and frustration in the survivor which may cause him or her to be very impatient. I am convinced it would be confusing to anyone who isn't a professional caregiver. Woe is the spouse who isn't able to absorb the oftentimes irrational behavior. It may be best to excuse one's self and leave the scene after fulfilling the survivor's request or putting the survivor to bed and making sure he or she is comfortable and safe. Sleep, with lots of rest, is the best tonic. Survivors, if like me, need an enormous amount of rest to rebuild their bodies. I was always tired. But one can, as the old saying goes, "enter into the trap of nature and fall in love with one's bed." The concern is never wanting to get out of bed. A regimen of rest, good diet, therapy, daily exercise, and getting out into the world seeing people is best. Having a calendar with a definite schedule is also important. "Write it down," I was properly reminded all the time.

For example, every Saturday for several months at 11 a.m., I was picked up by a friend and driven to the beach in a nearby town, Lake Worth. We would watch the bathers, the ocean, and together we would have lunch in a beachside restaurant I did not frequent before my stroke. Everything was new and different...no memories of my "old life."

That was good and that was important. I believe I had to ease into my new life with pleasant, cheerful experiences and leave my old life behind. For awhile, I avoided frequenting old haunts, old business associates, and refrained from any people or organizations that reminded me of previous controversies and business disappointments. I found myself gravitating to "what's good" and away from "what's not so good" — from everyone or anything that did not contribute to my healing.

I found the way out of my malaise and frequent depressions was to get outside of my daily world. Connecting with others was a major part of my emotional recovery. I made it a point to have someone, sometimes Ena, sometimes my friend Richard or cousins Rodney and Dudley, take me for rides or to lunch or dinner "out in the world." I felt awful sometimes, and so lonely at times. But I never quit. I am told these are typical emotional burdens stroke survivors must bear.

My life did get better. Nearly everyday I would be grateful as I spoke with God each morning, thankful that the day before had brought a new capability, a new awareness of the goodness of life. Prayer and my conversations with God were very comforting. And while progress and new abilities may not have been apparent every day, sometimes "two steps forward, one step back"...over a period of time I did sense progress. My cherished visitors would make me feel better when they would say, "Sandy, you've come a long way — you are standing straighter." Or, "Listening to you speak, I can't even tell you had a stroke. Your recovery is really amazing. Keep up the therapy."

Every month I received encouraging letters from the many friends in Japan I had made when I was chairman of the board of The Morikami Museum and Japanese Gardens. Two such correspondents, and dear friends, are Imai San and Mr. Toshio Tokuda, Mayor of the city of Miyazu, birthplace of George Morikami, the Japanese immigrant who settled in the Yamato colony between Delray Beach and Boca Raton in 1904. Mr. Morikami donated his 200 acres of farmland on which the museum is located to Palm Beach County. He was a dear friend of my father from 1924 until they both died in the late 1970s. Mayor Tokuda and I exchanged personal visits over several years, instituted student and teacher exchanges, and became good friends. That is why, after my stroke, when I received a letter from Mayor Tokuda, I would break out in tears, filled with emotion of our friendship. It's amazing how many times I would sit on my deck and read his letters, filled with "my friend, please make sure you focus on your therapy. It is the most important thing." They were wonderful.

Receiving his letters and letters from my other friends in Japan, including dear Mr. Toshinobu Wada, who was chairman of the board of the Japan Oil Exploration Corporation and lived in Tokyo, were among the most heartening and encouraging events for me. They reminded me that life and my world was greater than my bedroom, my living room and my terrace, which defined my world for many months after I came home.

Stubbornness is something else...sometimes to the point of becoming obsessive. It took on the very meaning of what I would do on frequent occasions. It meant grabbing hold of an issue and not "letting go" of it, thereby getting in the way of relief and moving on. For example, when I would lose something because I forgot where I put it, I had a terrible time. (This still happens sometimes because of my short-term memory loss.) But my stubbornness...compulsiveness?...would cause me to set aside almost every thought until I found whatever I misplaced. This was also true of getting a depressing issue in my mind, like remembering what I could do before my stroke and what I could not do now, ruminating over it all day long, silently letting it stay in the way, blocking all other helpful, positive thoughts. I found this happened when I was alone too much or very tired. Getting tired became a large part of my daily living because I consumed so much energy doing anything physical, like walking or, amazingly, simply pushing an elevator button with my left thumb (using virtually every muscle in the left side of my body from my leg to my shoulder and arm). I would get so very tired, and being tired, I would get caught in this trap of stubbornness. It takes time and effort to pull out of these places. But I am finally learning how to do that, although not completely as of yet. And my life has become a better, more fulfilling experience. It's not as though I don't have difficult times anymore. I still tire physically, but it happens less frequently and doesn't last as long these days.

Thank God I haven't lost my sense of humor. It keeps me from feeling morose when something doesn't "work" well. For instance, my left arm has uncontrollably responded very strangely to sharp sounds. When I hear a loud noise like thunder or when I yawn, my left arm spasms upward and hits me in the chin. I learned to laugh when I would yawn, expecting to be hit in my chin. Strange for sure, but even now, seven years later, it still reacts that way, though not as strongly. That too is part of left-sided neglect.

"My left hand always sits in my crotch," I would say, trying to get a laugh out of an embarrassing situation when friends would stop by. Then, when I stood up, my hand would automatically swing to "its position" in front of my crotch! So embarrassing, so funny actually...but beyond my control unless I consciously relocated my hand with my right hand! But then, sometimes it was good because I had forgotten to zip my pants and my left hand hid my error. So I made jokes about my hand having its own dirty mind. And I joked about putting some adversary's face under my chin and yawning several times to "bop" him in the face.

Coming home was a vital and major step in my recovery. Most of my life at home for several months was spent resting, reading, going to outpatient therapy at Pinecrest, sleeping, eating, and "letting go." It was a time of healing, of rest, of rebuilding, of renewal. I began to realize that I was starting the rest of my life anew. There were no expectations by anyone, including me. The obligations I carried, some by subconscious choice, no longer were mine. I tried to involve myself in family business affairs, but my own office had been closed down and all business had ceased. This, in itself, was a traumatic experience for me. Letting go of my career was devastating. At times I felt like a terrible burden on others and I sometimes felt a sense of guilt.

Yet, I was given a "new slate, a clear desk, and a plain sheet of paper," so to speak, on which to redefine my life, to begin again, to start over. Whether I felt negative thoughts vs. positive thoughts about the same subjects and felt either "bad" or "good" was very simply my attitude. That's all. That's the issue — one's view of life. We must choose the positive view and feel good, not bad. Still, I was grateful to be home.

One day when I was really miserable, my dear friend in California, Mimi Peak, told me over the telephone, "Sandy, look on this as a wonderful opportunity." At that time, I couldn't move...I couldn't help myself, and she's telling me this? Opportunity? Was she smoking funny stuff? But she was right! There were physical and mental difficulties to be sure. After all, I had been declared by the doctors to be permanently 100% disabled and there were good reasons for their deduction. That very statement caused me enormous emotional trauma. It was a horrible label that I had to learn to accept. It wasn't easy. It was very, very difficult for a long time. But I had a choice. I could feel angry and sorry for myself or I could somehow put the past behind me, begin again and do the very best I could with what God had given me. I could follow dear Mimi's advice and counsel or give up. Some use the *cliché* "play the cards I was dealt." I could stay in my home, live off my savings and some disability insurance, dwell in my own remorse and sadness, detach myself from the world and deteriorate emotionally and physically. Rather, I made a conscious decision to take a different path toward strength and independence. I enrolled in a therapy program to re-learn how to drive, overcome the stroke impact on my car insurance and begin to drive myself around town and re-enter the world. I found coming home opened up my awareness of many aspects of my life that were not part of my thought processes while I was in the hospital.

I also realized that the day would come when my 24-hour "live-in" would no longer be there. It was so easy to say, "Ena, I need a glass of water," or "Ena, when is dinner?" or "Ena, could you please adjust the thermostat?" I think I was getting very comfortable having a person who was happy to accommodate my every need. Certainly, I couldn't do much, especially at first. Getting out of a chair after putting on my left leg brace, then straining mentally and physically to stand up, finding my cane, slowly and carefully taking my first step, and avoiding with great deliberation any obstacle to finally reach the kitchen or the thermostat was exhausting. I often dropped my cane on the ground and had to struggle to pick it up…that's why there are four-legged canes. Obstacles like a chair or table were of major concern. I knew if my left foot (I still had left-toe drop) were to catch a leg of a table or some other fixed object, I would lose my balance and, sometimes, fall onto the floor.

So, rather than go through all that effort and accept that risk, I would ask Ena to do all sorts of favors and duties for me. But I knew, and rarely forgot, the sometimes depressing and sometimes happy thoughts that soon I would (if I could) fend for myself. I would resume cooking for myself, taking care of myself, making my own bed, going to the bathroom and performing all my hygienic duties for myself and taking showers alone, without a chair on which to sit. These normal activities that we all take for granted were not available to me, but rather they were goals, objectives and dreams that one day I would resume doing. One day…

After having stayed with me 24 hours a day for five months, Ena moved on. After she departed, I had an opportunity to take in a male roommate who would reside in my guestroom as had Ena, and would cook for me, clean, and be my aide. I spoke to Rebecca about this. She was adamantly opposed. So I stayed alone as she urged and found she was absolutely correct. I have been told that I progressed better and faster because I lived alone.

My occupational therapist had helped me learn the activities of daily living (ADL) and had provided exercises for me from the waist up, i.e., my arms and upper body. Such confidence-building tasks included bathing and dressing myself, making my bed, doing my laundry, carrying my full laundry basket with both hands, cooking, cleaning, sweeping with a broom and the like. These are important ways of building self-esteem and should be undertaken even if they are very difficult and intimidating. Today I am virtually self-assured in my hygiene activities, thanks to my occupational therapy.

After Ena left, Joy, a lovely nursing assistant, came to see me three days each week as I transitioned over time to a place when I would soon be alone full time. She didn't stay over like Ena, and for the first time I was alone after dinner. To be sure, it was emotionally difficult to accept their departures. It was sad because Ena and I had grown close and it was a bit scary letting go. It was the same emotional "tug" I had felt when I first came home from the hospital. Joy became so important to my life because she was the bridge between dependence and independence.

When Joy came, and I was a bit stronger, she would talk with me, show me ways to continue to improve my daily life. As a result, I became aware of what are called *enhancements*. *Enhancement* is the word given to those tools, which are available by catalog, that help people who cannot use both hands have an easier time performing routine tasks and thus enable them to get along without constant assistance. There are many types of enhancements — a special cutting board, top opener, rocker knife for cutting with one hand, right hand can opener, button hooks, etc.

For instance, when I need to open a jar or bottle, I grab it with my right hand and place it into the fixed gadget screwed in place under the bottom of the upper cabinet in my kitchen. After placing the cap in the appropriate place, I twist the bottle and *voila*! — a loose cap! There is also a one-handed electric can opener in my kitchen.

Washing both hands with a bar of soap is not an option since my left hand stays open or clenched. So, I use a small fingernail cleaning brush with two suction cups to hold it in place in my sink. My shoelaces have been replaced with Velcro, the magical miracle of the decade.

Even though I use a clipboard to hold my writing pad in place, I learned, clumsily at first, — at the urging of Rebecca, my "therapist emeritus"— to also place my left hand on the pad. That is how I write letters, sign checks, address envelopes, and eventually wrote the manuscripts of my first book, and indeed, most of this book. Learning to use my left hand to hold the paper pad in place took time, but improved my healing.

After a few months I began my driving therapy. It was a bit scary at first, but the therapist was very helpful and patient. It was similar to driver education, with dual controls and extra training to compensate for the primary use of one hand, arm and leg. Lucky for me my right foot was controllable for the accelerator and brake pedal. During the early lessons I tightly gripped the wheel, scared I might hit someone. I was taut, stiff, and unsure of myself. It reminded me of the first time I tried snow skiing, water-skiing or driving at 16...I was very nervous and clenched. I was in totally unfamiliar territory even though I had been driving for years. After about six months, as I continued my other outpatient physical and occupational therapies, I accomplished a major victory. I could now drive myself whenever and wherever I chose. My newly gained sense of accomplishment and freedom from being able to drive again and attend happy events like concerts, street fairs, and church was instrumental in restoring my independence and ease around other people. Determination and commitment to work hard each day was absolutely necessary to regain my independence. The more I did so, in little steps, the more I could adjust to my new life and not get angry or frustrated. It wasn't easy, far from it. It was hard for me.

I found that each day I gained more confidence and accomplished more and more. I felt as if I was building a huge earthen dam, one stone at a time. I began to realize that I was rebuilding my self-esteem by building confidence. And building confidence in myself was vitally important. That could only be attained by staying on a course of accomplishment, rejoining my world, seeing my friends and socializing.

After six months of outpatient physical therapy, I was told "that's all we can do for you." But though I walked with a cane, I knew I didn't walk as well as I wanted or as well as I had after three months with Rebecca. I still wore the leg brace. I hitched my hip and slung my left leg outward. I was always off balance. My left knee snapped at every step. It was hard and painful all the time. And they were saying, "That's all we can do." I would not believe that. I knew there was more to do. Yet, the hospital was, in their view, finished. Was it the insurance company limits? Three

months later, my outpatient occupational therapists.
said, "We can't do any more with your arm. Two more
sessions is all we can do for you." I was prepared to pay
if that was the issue, but they wouldn't say.

My hospital-based physical and occupational
therapy was coming to an end. Yet, I knew I had much
more to do and more to gain. I could hardly move my
left arm the slightest bit and couldn't feel a thing, and
they were saying, "We can't do anymore for your arm."
That was very depressing. I was not going to stop here,
but where was I to go? Suddenly, I felt abandoned,
unsure and alone. When you've lost your self-
confidence and self-esteem, uncertainty becomes very
much a threat. You have to get rid of the sad feelings,
get determined and find another way.

As I was leaving one of my last outpatient
sessions at the hospital, I saw my friend Kurt, brother-
in-law of Elsie, a fellow outpatient, who encouraged me
to go to a local, private therapy clinic that he said had a
good reputation.

A bit discouraged but hopeful, the next day I
went to the clinic he had suggested.

"If I walk a few steps for you, can you please
tell me if you can help me?" I asked.

Ray, the therapist that I had heard such good
things about, said, "Walk to me."

I did, using a cane, hitching my hip and slinging
my left leg still wearing a brace. My toes on my left
foot would "claw," causing constant, severe pain. I
ultimately had them straightened surgically.

Ray watched me and said, "Yes, I can help
you."

I was very happy, smiled and then broke into
tears when he told me, "We'll have that brace off your
leg in six weeks."

I replied, "But they said I may have to wear it for years and I hate it. I hate having to put it on and take it off just to go to the bathroom."

Sure enough, six weeks later, the brace came off and I felt like a bird in flight. I was now back to where I was when I left Rebecca.

I spent one hour, three days each week with Ray. After nearly two years of ice rubbings with vibration and electric shocks on my left limbs by his terrific assistants and instructions from my new therapist, I was steadily rejoining the human race.

Biofeedback sessions and continuing physical therapy are essential in bringing back weak side capabilities. I remember the day I showed off for my cousin Nancy, who always smiled when she saw me — so warm, so loving, so encouraging. I showed her how I could, for the first time, turn the doorknob with my left hand and open the door. After an initial struggle, I finally was able to flip on the light switch with my left hand. It took enormous effort, using most of the muscles on my left side as my confused brain turned on most of my muscles by mistake. My counter muscles were straining, working against each other, tiring me whenever I tried anything with my left arm or leg. I was exhausted, and it took several minutes to do each task. Then, I pressed the elevator button for Nancy, again showing off what I could do with my left hand — the hand the doctors thought I would never use again. I was dripping with perspiration and very tired as muscle fought muscle. My hand was spastic and moved everywhere but toward the button, and my left shoulder would strain upward as my muscles fought each other without any coordination. But what an achievement! Every seemingly small step was a major victory. Each took tremendous effort and all my mental concentration and focus to achieve each of these simple tasks we all take for granted.

I constantly heard from therapists and my doctors who were surprised with how far I had come. They thought that my significant improvement was astounding and inspirational to others — a "miracle in progress." Each time I heard that, I felt compelled to encourage other stroke "victors," as we call each other.

My first experience encouraging others occurred when I was asked to meet with Kurt's sister-in-law, a recent stroke patient. Elsie, age 75, was very depressed and angry at having suffered her stroke. When I found her in the hospital corridor,. she was sitting in her wheelchair, slumped over, and crying, surrounded by members of her loving family. I offered her counseling. She understood and, being of strong German heritage, became emotionally empowered. With wonderful support from her family, especially her son Herb and brother-in-law Kurt, Elsie steadfastly pursued her therapy. Like many of us, she improved steadily, slowly, sometimes with plateaus and sometimes with what seemed to be setbacks. We would joke about our progress. She had that indomitable "can do — must do" spirit. She and her family have become dear friends of mine. Elsie has never given up and still, now in her eighties, continues her therapy in order to improve her ability to function independently.

By my sixth month, as an outpatient, I attended and participated in monthly stroke support group meetings at both hospitals where I gave and received support from other stroke survivors. I strongly recommend attending stroke support group meetings. I had significantly reduced my involvement in parts of my former world by leaving some boards of directors of businesses and civic organizations. It's good to pick and choose those places, events, and people that make one feel good about oneself. Avoid conflict, stressful situations, and reminders of bad feelings. It became a matter of being very careful to be around those people who enhanced my life, who gave me unconditional love and encouragement. I involved myself in new groups with new interests to me and I gave what I could. And it began to make all the difference. I loved seeing people and, looking back, it was to my great advantage not to be concerned with "how I looked to myself or to others." After coming home, I began ridding myself of the feeling of having to measure up to anyone else's opinion. This was a new experience for me. For years I was always conscious of either being someone's son or brother or having expectations placed on me by others and by myself. But now I was starting over with my new life, with no obligations, no responsibilities and no mental obstacles. Only smooth sailing albeit with my new impairments.

I was now back home and slowly moving toward a sense of *acceptance*. I found that I could revisit downtown, see friends, be friendly and pleasant to those who had been opposed to me in my business efforts and had caused me so much grief. I believe my newfound and growing sense of well-being was becoming evident to myself and to others. I was now a stroke survivor, no longer in the real estate development business, and though physically impaired, my mind was, thank God, as capable as before my stroke. While, like most severe stroke survivors, I now needed a cane, dragged my left leg and had a flaccid left arm in front of me, I was mentally, but not yet emotionally, equal to my prior condition. From my view, I was not impaired because I was able to put behind me the fact that I had had a stroke by detaching myself from the physical impairments and reattaching myself to my world. It required acceptance and the comfort of home. In many ways, I began to act like my "old self."

My progress during the next few years was astounding. I found that I progressed much faster having to do things for myself as opposed to having someone wait on me and cater to my needs. When I visited the private therapy clinic, made excellent gains in the way I walked, associated with the therapists, and nurtured my sense of humor, I felt better about myself. I came to realize that "therapy" was a word that could and must apply to the entire person, whether learning how to control my walk or arm use, mouth symmetry or sensations of feeling on my left side or, indeed, how I saw the world. It requires healing of the total person, not just the physical.

It seemed I was achieving a good balance in my life. While I devoted myself to my "therapeutic experience," I had rejoined the world socially by painting and writing.

In time, I came to realize I could do without those interests in my life before my stroke, like quasi-government or business boards.

I found that everyone I met was kind to me. My minister, Rev. Donald Clauson, had told me in the hospital when I had angrily asked him, "Where is God anyway?" He had said, "He is everywhere, and you will see Him in other people as they extend their love and kindness to you." He was so right, and I've been reminded of his wisdom every day.

Still, there were reminders of activities I really enjoyed before my stroke and wished I could do again. For example, on Sundays I had enjoyed riding my bicycle along the beach, loving the seascapes, casually greeting people and peddling to homes of friends. I also looked forward to my Saturdays, weather permitting, of sailing my Hobie Cat offshore and racing the flying fish my sailboat would stir out of the water. "Flying" across the ocean just inches above the waves, experiencing the breezes in my face, smelling the sea, entertaining my one or two passengers, and feeling the close relationship with the ocean's waves was exhilarating.

Now, I had to face the fact, the reality, that I could not ride my bicycle or sail my Cat. I couldn't push the boat down to the sea or even walk on the soft sand of the beach that "gave" under my feet without falling down.

My life *was* different, and I *had* to accept this new reality, or become miserably frustrated, angry, and unpleasant. I chose the former, not the latter. And it made the difference in my view of life, enabling me to appreciate other things, like the colors in the sky, the people I meet, and so many other blessings. I knew too that I had changed, and maybe my new view of the world was attracting people. I could feel a new sense of purpose, a new spirituality, and I liked it.

Chapter 5

It's All In The Mind

What you visualize, you can actualize

Where there is no vision, the
people perish.
Proverbs 29:18

The solution to overcoming the terrible damage
from a stroke requires a positive attitude, a vision, and a
sense of determination, all of which are available to us
if we will just use them. It's all in the mind.

A stroke is an attack on the brain, which is the
locale of our mind. Therefore, it is safe to say that the
place where the injury occurred, the brain, is also the
place where the solution is located. We can, for sure,
agree that the mind is where we find our attitudes,
whether they be optimism, pessimism, determination,
faith, hope, eagerness, sense of futility, sadness, anger
— all our emotions. We create fantasies, visions and
perceptions in our mind.

And this is the point, the essence of this chapter
and of the healing process which, ultimately, leads to
acceptance, the final stage in the cycle of grief. We can
draw on the wisdom of our doctors and instructions
from our therapists. But how we use that information to

regain our lives depends on our own attitude. The classic steps in the cycle of grief that accompany any major crisis we all face in life are:

Denial: This can't be happening! What is happening to my body? This has to be a horrible nightmare from which I will awaken.

Depression: How am I going to live with this? I am so lonely and feel so abandoned and separated from God and everyone I know. I can't do *anything* for myself.

Anger: Why is this happening to me? I am angry with God. Where is he?

Bargaining: I try to minimize the extent of the damage in my mind and to hold on desperately to my life before the stroke.

Acceptance: I slowly began to reach an inner peace and enlightenment through prayer, and my creative potential through painting and writing.

I came to realize that there was only one way to begin the healing process. I had to accept my new life, who I was, what had happened to me, take responsibility for my life, and commit to making the best of a bad situation. I had to create my own vision of my life, create my own reality, seek God's strength and determination and get on with it. I felt I had to have this breakthrough, this total and complete shift in my way of thinking. My life before was done...history. Sad, but true. Letting go of my life was and still is extremely difficult. Many stroke survivors are never able to accomplish this vital step. In some cases that I am familiar with, they remain sad, depressed, and unable to become active again. They give up, wallow in self-pity and deteriorate, and never walk again or go out of their homes. They must be encouraged as much as possible to adjust their thinking and find meaningful reasons to strive toward living a better life.

And so, as I began my therapies in earnest, I began to develop a new attitude. I created my own reality of where I hoped I would go, where I felt I must go, and finally, where I was *determined* to go. All of this attitudinal change had to come from my mind, my brain. I am, and always have been, convinced that as Dale Carnegie said, "Of 100 high school graduates, essentially all nearly equal in health, intelligence, and physical condition, only five by age 65 will be self-supporting and independent. Those five will succeed because of one ingredient that sets them apart. That ingredient is *attitude*."

Imagine, only five of 100. That means 95 will not. Some will be on charity, and some will be financially or emotionally unable to cope. Attitude is the single ingredient that defines their future. Attitude is what determines our success at overcoming a stroke's terrible impact on our lives. The impact is overtly physical to be sure, but I am convinced that the emotional impact is as severe. Most, if not all, stroke survivors suffer depression, some severely. That depression can be permitted to linger and get worse or it can be reduced or turned around. We can deal with our emotions and we can find help to accomplish this. It is not easy and the solution does not arrive adequately for all stroke survivors. However, I believe, coming from as deep a depression and from as severe a brain injury as I experienced, other stroke survivors can overcome much, if not all, of their depression and anger. They must receive good medical, psycho-physical, occupational therapies, and nurturing from their friends and family. They need a sense of purpose, of being needed.

My Aunt Mary is 89 years old and still in her wheelchair twelve years after her life threatening ischemic stroke. It struck the left hemisphere and paralyzed her right side. Being right-handed, her writing, eating and other activities had to be transferred to her left hand.

Aunt Mary suffers significant impairments from her stroke. She can speak, but suffers from a type of aphasia (difficulty in connecting words). She has to spend quite a bit of time at "word-search." When Aunt Mary says an incorrect word, she adds, "Wait a minute, I'll get it," or sometimes, in frustration, "Later." She corrects herself with a laugh when she forgets names, even those of her children or grandchildren. She doesn't get angry. Sometimes, she'll call me on the phone and instead of saying, "Hello," she'll start with "Goodbye." She will also forget my name or confuse it with someone else. When she is ready to hang up, she'll laugh and say, "Hello."

Aunt Mary had a very spiritual upbringing. Her father, my grandfather, was a priest in the Antiochian Eastern Orthodox Church. He taught us almost daily all our lives. Aunt Mary, like her sisters and brothers, including my mother, were imbued with the belief that faith can accomplish anything and that it is better to be happy than sad.

Aunt Mary was a "flapper girl" in her youth and loved to dance. I once asked her, "Aunt Mary, what was a flapper girl anyway?" She broke into a broad smile, snapped her fingers, as though she was listening to her own orchestra (she does this often as she rocks her shoulders to music), and said, "Hot stuff!"

Today Aunt Mary is in her wheelchair most of the day. Kay, a wonderful, caring 24-hour live-in aide, cooks and tends to her needs. Aunt Mary attends church every Sunday at the 8:00 a.m. service. Her nephews, son and spouses in turn attend to be with her. After church, we all get together for a scrumptious breakfast at Ellie's, our favorite retreat. It's a 1950s style local restaurant owned and operated by our friends Ellie and Bob.

Aunt Mary has always known how to live, how to enjoy life. Everytime I greet her I ask, "How are you today, Aunt Mary?" "I feel great" is always her response. I once asked her how she can love her life in spite of her impairments — unable to walk or use her hands, cook, feed herself or tend to her bathroom needs. Her reply was, "Life is too precious and I'm not about to give it up! I am taking therapy again and will get even better. It's all in your mind. Where there is life, there is hope. And I believe where there is hope, there can be faith." With this attitude, the mind is positive and optimistic, and can focus on healing emotionally and physically.

Aunt Mary is certainly testimony to a winning attitude. She has now learned to feed herself, using her left hand to hold the fork. This is quite a feat for her. We all go to see her regularly because she is so upbeat, so much fun. If she wallowed in self-pity, I feel sure she would be unhappy and fewer people would want to be with her. Aunt Mary is aware of her conditions, and yet, stays cheery, and still corrects us when we need it. She lives with joy and empowerment. I find myself going to see her often. And I feel good. Actually, I get as much or more out of our discussions as she does. She remains an inspiration to me. She encourages me to "pass on the joy of life."

Are there times when I am unhappy? Of course. Some mornings I know I have to get up, yet I don't want to. Sometimes I am angry, depressed and frustrated. But I've learned not to let those feelings last long. This is very typical and should be expected after a stroke.

There are several things I have grown accustomed to accepting, another key creation of the mind, and that is, I must do my stretching, my weight bearing and the like as regularly as I eat my meals for the rest of my life. But so what? Acceptance is a wonderful state of mind — so is determination, hope and faith. These are all vital characteristics that must be found and adopted as part of our being...our healing.

I have found that whatever I can do or think that makes me feel better about myself is good. Rebuilding and sustaining a healthy sense of self-esteem and self-image is a must.

My friend Roy, 70, who suffered a left side stroke, walks very well and his right arm paralysis went away within six weeks, but he has aphasia. He cannot remember anyone's name, even those of people he has known for years and sees often. He cannot identify numbers either. If you raise two fingers, he cannot tell that it is "two." He has to count from one, like a child learns. Yet, his wife, Betty, hastens to add, "But, he reconciles his bank statement each month." As Roy laughs at his own situation, he will say, "It's a fascinating experience." During football season, he'll raise two fingers high and chuckle while exclaiming, "We're number one!" He has learned to accept his post-stroke changes, remain humorous, and enjoy his life. I am sure he feels frustration at times, but he's healing wonderfully. I have known Roy over 50 years. Even today, when we meet and I say, "Hi, Roy," he will respond, "Hi, quick, tell me your name." He may or may not remember my name a few moments after I tell him, so I repeat my name several times during our conversation, with a smile matching his.

Knowing that the healing process never ends and that therapy continues to help me get better is empowering, and gives me good reasons for continued determination. It becomes a way of life. It's different, and could easily be frustrating, which it is sometimes. So is the summer heat, but what are you going to do about it?

Actually, therapy can be fun. For example, with the help of a physical therapist, there is aqua therapy which is very helpful, pleasurable and soothing and keeps the muscles and joints toned and responsive. Depending on one's financial position, it can be done at the public pool, at the clinic, the pool at one's home, apartment complex, or on a cruise ship around the world. What better place to spend some of your disposable income than on rehabilitating one's health? Why not? Like the joke about a wealthy deceased person's will being read by the attorney, "Being of sound mind, I spent it all."

As much as possible, three times a week, I go to the gym for stretching and to improve my cardiovascular needs by bicycle riding therapy. People there are concerned about their own health and are friendly, lively, helpful and understanding. I see friendly faces, get back into the world and make new friends. I laugh a lot, make jokes, and enjoy making others laugh. Try it, it's great medicine.

I recommend a personally prescribed, doctor-supervised program that will help your progress by specifically taking on those workouts that will foster improvement. I must avoid heavy muscle building because it creates more "tone" in my muscle and can make it difficult for me to walk properly. These gym sessions also boost my self-esteem by building body strength.

I dare not too get comfortable; I dare instead to get uncomfortable so I will produce favorable results. I dare to dream. I dare to be enthusiastic and to seek new ways to heal myself, again with God's help, emotionally, culturally, and physically. Two out of three isn't all bad. Soon, it will be "three for three."

I know the best is yet to come and I know for that to happen I must nurture my positive attitude, look ahead and say " good-bye and thank you" to my old life and say "hello" to my new life. Each day I know I must take action to take me to a place I've never been before. I remind myself more of what I can do, and less and less of what I cannot do. It is very difficult, but it is possible — and it's becoming easier every day. It is a lot like eating an elephant: only one bite at a time. It's too big a challenge unless you take it step by step, or one bite at a time. You cannot eat the entire elephant at one sitting. And you cannot overcome the terrible damages of a stroke in a day or month. It takes time, lots of time. But most of all, it takes the enormous power of the mind. In fact, *it's all in the mind.* And, one day, as I have found, a stroke survivor is able to say, "Thank you, God, for allowing the healing to begin almost immediately. Thank you, God, for giving me the power of my mind to bring all the powers of the universe to bear, to help me, heal me, my body and my mind."

When I was in the hospital, my brothers, and Nancy, my cousin, assumed the responsibility of picking up the pieces of my life by shutting down my office and deciding what should be disposed of, getting my books in order, writing checks and paying bills. During the first month or two, they would ask my approval to sell my sailboat (with the assumption implicit that I would never be able to sail again), sell my car (with the assumption that I would never drive again) and vacate my offices by removing all furniture, files and paintings (preparing for the likelihood that I would never resume my business career). It was a difficult time for me emotionally because it emphasized harshly that my old life was gone. I was trying to hang on to that life as much as I could.

But it was very difficult for them too. They really came to my rescue. They were being realistic, especially since they were more aware of my condition than was I. So, I acquiesced on most requests, trying to stay only a bit involved in the decision-making. They were wonderful. They took up the reins and visited me often, especially on Sunday afternoons. Sometimes we would sit outside on the terrace. They sat in chairs around the umbrella-covered table and I was in my wheelchair.

They would always bring me news of family, friends, and our community.

"Ernie," I recall saying to my oldest brother as the others listened, "I promise you I *will walk* down Atlantic Avenue." (I was speaking of the main street of our town, Delray Beach.) Setting achievable goals was my best incentive to expand my capabilities and to reinforce and sustain my hope to the turn to the full use of them.

"You will do that, Sandy. That's a do-able goal. You *have* to do that, Sandy," he replied.

Recalling that moment, I realize we were both responding to our father and mother's teaching to call on all our courage, determination and tenacity with an absolute responsibility we must assume to do whatever was necessary to overcome whatever adversity had befallen us. Our parents had always shown that determination: "Son, in life things are going to happen to you; some will be very bad and make your life miserable. But it's not so much about what happens to you that determines who you are. Rather, who you are is determined by how you behave under those circumstances, how you respond. Never give in. You must overcome these difficulties." And so it was. I knew I had to do whatever I had to do to walk by myself down our main street. When? Who knew? Timing wasn't an issue. But there I had my confirmation from Ernie who spoke, and from Roy and Charlie who both nodded and smiled, affirming we had the same genes and upbringing. We had the same attitudes toward life.

Walking under my own power was the symbol of victory. Walking downtown meant I wanted to *and would* rejoin my friends and fellow townspeople, especially at the local popular diner, my favorite, The Green Owl on Atlantic Avenue (our version of "Cheers — where everyone knows your name"). So, I had a perfect vision of my goal. Something clear was in my mind. Something measurable, defined, simple. It was, to me, like a crossbar for a high jumper, the finish line for a dash runner, a goal line for a football player.

When I was in the twelfth month following my stroke, after intensive and arduous therapy, Richard, my cousin and life-long friend, came to pick me up at my apartment. We went to the family store he and his sister-in-law, Alice, operated across the street from The Green Owl.

I called my brothers and told them, "I'm with Richard at the store. Please come over if you can. It's been a year and I'm going to walk, without assistance, down the street to the bank and then back to The Green Owl for lunch. I want you to be with me."

Unfortunately, Charlie was solidly booked with appointments in his dental offices. Ernie and Roy, whose offices were a few blocks away, came to the store. They walked with me during one of the greatest, most wonderful, exhilarating and victorious moments of my life. I had walked again! *Downtown!* Not just in the therapy gym!

That was a heady experience and gave me enormous confidence and courage to work harder. Though I still retained a "limp," and I was fatigued several times and had to rest, I knew I was on the right path to freedom and independence. But there was more, much more to do. The best part is that my mind was in control of my body again. At least the parts that enabled me to walk. What I had set as a goal, what I had visualized, had been actualized. Yes, it is *all in the mind.*

Chapter 6

The Path To Healing

Stroke survivors want desperately to go back to what they knew, what was comfortable, what was familiar. I now realize that wanting what you *cannot* have is an empty pursuit. What you *can* have is time! It is the time to rest, to think and to be without obligations, responsibilities — it can also be the time of opportunity — the time for healing.

I guess you learn the most when you are suffering the most. In fact, had it not been for the stroke, I would never have entered my creative career in writing and painting. During much of our lives, we create in our minds a painting of ourselves predicated on what we think we should or should not do and what we believe others might think of us or want us to be. We are greatly influenced by our parents, peers and the society in which we live, or, at least, by our *perception* of their opinions.

Many of us stroke survivors are not willing to be seen in public with our infirmities because we believe we would appear to be a lesser person in the eyes of our contemporaries, our audiences. This is also true about people who have recently divorced, suffered significant   financial   setbacks   and   the   like.

Embarrassment and undue concern about what others may think is a very human response. But it is a miserable trap and serves to inhibit or even prohibit the healing process that should be occurring. Rather, we must learn to simply *be* who we are to be. We must "listen to our heart" and "march to our own drummer." It is true that we are each unique and have a singular life to live.

We are regrettably most concerned with our physical impairments in large part because we are afraid that the world will see us as *less* than we were before. We *know*, we absolutely *believe*, that the stroke has made us physically less than we were, and therefore we are lesser persons. We do not believe our life after the stroke can be better in any conceivable way. We know it will surely be different, meaning *worse*. If, at the time I was in the hospital, someone told me my new life was going to be *different*, I would have interpreted that to mean *less*. That is because I would have been focused on my impaired, therefore *less*, "physical self." Yet, I was taught in my religion that focusing on one's self was contrary to God's wishes. I am also convinced now that in spite of a good deal of residual physical impairment, my new life is much better in many ways. I have been able to disregard almost completely my fear of what others might perceive me to be. It is truly wonderful to be relieved from a self-imposed, very heavy emotional burden.

Before true healing can take place though, a shift in one's perception of self must occur. From a spiritual viewpoint, focusing only on the physical aspects of life is an   unrewarding path. Rather, even in a secular sense, one must not perceive the physical impairments as a measure of one's value as a member of society. Changing one's perception of one's self is a means to grow spiritually closer to God who made us and loves us. It is a means to heal culturally, emotionally, intellectually and spiritually. If this healing takes place, one develops a new and stronger capability to envision one's new reality. By focusing on one's mental and emotional healing, one can become empowered with enormous faith and positive vision. In this way, the physical impairments can more likely be corrected and overcome. The reverse is also true. If one cannot overcome depression, anger or sadness, the physical healing will be significantly hindered and the symbiotic relationship between emotional and physical healing and improvements cannot take place.

Thus, the survivor, his loved ones, caregivers and therapists, who are all participating in the healing process, should encourage, support and advise one another by emphasizing the spiritual, physiological and emotional therapeutic effects.

I was carefully instructed to rest, rest, rest. Those periods of rest and "quiet time" were also times of thought and emotional healing.

I desperately wanted to walk again, become physically independent and rejoin my world as a productive member of society *on my terms*. During the five months Ena was with me, following my three months of intensive therapy at Pinecrest Rehabilitation Hospital, she pushed me in my wheelchair while I met with dedicated counselors. I slowly learned not to feel too self-conscious, probably because I was receiving so much kindness and friendliness from everyone. No one shied away or turned their heads. The fear of others' opinions was not part of my thinking during those months.

By my seventh month, I was walking short distances with a cane and leg brace. I didn't walk with "beauty" — my left leg slung out to the side, my hip would lift, and my left arm was in my crotch as usual! I was in poor posture whether bent over and looking down, or leaning backward. Both postures were reflective of my body's lack of coordination. I did my best to ignore my "imperfections," but I was sad to believe this might be my destiny. When I walked by a mirror or store window, which reflected like a mirror, I saw how clumsily I walked, and how "different" I was from others. I harshly judged myself and became my own "worst critic." So, I quit looking at mirrors and reflective shop windows. That was my solution.

Yet, somehow, I was happy that I *could* walk downtown, and I learned not to be concerned about what others might think. Nor did I consider how I would handle their well-meaning sympathetic greetings that came my way. Sometimes one has to propel oneself to break loose of remembering what one could do, but now cannot do. It's a slow process.

Over time, I reached deeply into my spiritual oasis to get into silent and peaceful communication with God. I prayed every morning before I did anything else. I thanked God for all His blessings, even listing those blessings each day to remind myself of how God loved me and would not leave me.

As I look back, these lists usually began with "thank you God for my good health." I was in my wheelchair as I wrote the first of these many "blessing lists" looking outward toward the sky, the ocean, the trees. It doesn't matter what you are gazing at as you thank God, for He is indeed everywhere. One only has to seek Him and listen.

I included the blessings of anything and everything that I *could* do. For example, I could *see* the beauty of the clouds, I could *hear* the birds in the sky, I could *feel* the soft breezes, I could *smell* the flowers, and I could *touch* the faces of my visitors. I was surrounded by beautiful creations of God.

Other legal pads became full of lists of "happy words"...those that best described God's presence. Words like rainbow, butterfly, full moon, sunrise...words that made me feel good. Sometimes I would fill pages of a ledger with hundreds of these "happy words."

Every Saturday morning, for months, Ted and Gloria, my friends from Atlanta, would call me on the telephone to find out how I was doing, encourage me and boost my spirits. If I was sad or down, Ted would say, "Get out your legal pad and let's write down all your blessings and the good things in your life." Afterward, he would ask me, "How do you feel now?"

I was reminded of all these wonders that I didn't take time to notice before my stroke when I was on my own gerbil wheel seeking to satisfy the self-imposed needs and expectations of society, and not my emotional or spiritual needs. It is critically important that the patient/survivor walk this path of enlightenment. This is the healing path that, if chosen, enables the survivor to convert this terrible experience into a new, better approach to life.

Discipline, I have found, must be used to overcome the constant yearning to give up, to stay in bed, to do nothing. It is an enormous requirement, but one *must* achieve a sense of positiveness.

Bill Bradley, in his 1999 presidential campaign, while reflecting on his years as a successful basketball star, spoke about "the personal discipline it takes to be positive."

In order to live a life of good feeling, optimism and hope, it is vital that each of us devote ourselves to the monumental task of being and feeling positive. It takes enormous discipline and courage to overcome the ever-present reminders that our lives after a severe stroke are a shadow of what our lives were before our stroke. But that can be done. In the hospital, I found everything around me reminded me that I was in deep trouble and my life would be "different." Doctors and nurses did everything they could to help me, but those very actions and behavior never let me forget that I was the patient, that I needed help, assistance and encouragement all the time. Visitors, loved ones and friends, by their very presence, reminded me I was unable to fully take care of myself like I could, and did, only a few days earlier.

My continuing process reinforces my courage to think positively and to continue my therapeutic exercises. Sometimes it takes courage just to get out of bed! And that means it's up to me to develop and maintain a positive, optimistic attitude filled with faith even when I *don't* want to do my exercises or therapy. All stroke survivors go through this daily test.

The other option, I am convinced, is more "hell on earth." And this form of hell is both clearly physical *and* mental. The anguish can be severe. As the mental attitude becomes more and more negative, the physical capability follows suit and the reverse is absolutely true also. My inability to comfortably stand, walk, and go down or up stairs or ramps constantly reminds me of my impairment, and that reminder impacts on my ability to think hopefully and positively — *if I let it* — which I cannot do.

It's hard to ask others to do for me those things I used to do without help...yet, as I have become more and more aware, I am more a "passenger" and not in charge (a control freak?). I am learning to feel comfortable asking others to help me or to do things for me. It's still not easy for me. For a long time, I yielded to the urge to prefer doing without instead of accepting help or favors. Now I realize that others *want* to help. And now, as part of my emotional healing, it is easier for me to see help from others as their gift to me, and I am getting better at accepting their personal gifts.

I recall twice in one month going to the beach. I had taken a few steps on the sand before, and felt sure I could do it again. But this time, the beach sand was very soft and my left foot twisted into an exaggerated way so that I was nearly walking on the outside of my ankle. Of course I fell down. Strangers rushed to help me up. Happily, kindness is all around us, and often, even before I ask for help, strangers leap to my assistance. I know I'm on my healing path when I graciously thank them.

When I get self-focused and down, I become aware of how miserable I am to myself and to my caregivers by giving them an added burden. When it's so depressing, I fight not to allow my mind to "go there." I always have to remind myself: "You *can* get better" and "yo*u can* do it." My twin mantras.

As I write, I am reminded that it has been more than six years since I suffered my stroke. I am still acutely aware of those physical activities I cannot now do that I did before. Some I miss, like snow skiing, water skiing, sailing and mountain climbing. Other activities I miss are playing tennis, tying shoe laces, hanging my trousers on a hangar without wrinkling the fabric, and tying a tie around my neck. (Before my stroke, I could tie a Windsor knot in one minute flat.) I cannot yet move quickly, or run, swim or jog, or join my brother and friends for a round of 18 holes on the golf course.

I am also becoming more aware of what I *can* do that I didn't do well before, like *not* wear a tie around my neck, writing, relaxing, painting, and being empathetic with just about everyone who comes into my life.

I loved to play golf and feel the club head make contact with that little white ball. What a feeling! For a long time, I thought I would never experience that sensation again. But I was wrong. Now, after lessons, getting out there and trying, I can. And I do. And now that I can, my mental attitude has gotten so much more positive and confident. As a result, my physical and emotional healing continue to improve. I prefer the positive approach and encourage every survivor to do likewise. I was committed and determined to get back on the golf course even if I couldn't hit the ball as far as before my stroke and could use only my right arm. I'm able to play pretty good golf, although three or four holes are about my physical limit. And I have more fun doing it! I think that's because I have had to become more realistic with my expectations. It's getting better all the time as I rebuild my stamina and endurance.

Sure, everything I do is harder and takes longer than before my stroke...even the simplest things. I find I consume enormous amounts of energy no matter what I do. Walking is a chore, and when I must walk anywhere, I preplan where I'm going, how I'm going to navigate around obstacles like furniture, and map the shortest route. I subconsciously understand I don't want to do it twice. It's just too tiring.

Dressing myself is still a chore. The hardest things used to be the easiest, like buttoning my shirts and trousers. I find that darned button inside my trousers is the hardest, causing me to twist my body. Of course, losing a few pounds in my middle would help a lot too! As for my shoes, I've gone to loafers or sneakers with Velcro. Shoelaces are not in the cards. There are available elastic shoelaces that tied once look good and the shoes then become a laced pair of "loafers." I find my attitude has changed from easy anger and frustration to finding better solutions. The sense of being overwhelmed has dissipated.

My therapist reminds me, "Use your left hand if you ever want to learn! If you don't, if you continue to neglect your left side limbs, they won't become part of your consciousness. Do more weight bearing and you'll be able to hold your left hand flat." As I do, my personal discipline grows and evolves into more confidence. Then my sense of positiveness grows too. It becomes a multiplier effect that accelerates the healing process. Success begets success begets confidence.

If I want things done, like keeping my bed made and shaving each day, and keeping my spirits up, I must do them myself. I am reminded of the emotional courage and esteem of the prisoners of war in the Academy Award winner *The Bridge on the River Kwai*, "stiff upper lip and all that British discipline." (They shaved and dressed properly every day in spite of their imprisonment.) It *does* keep your sense of self-esteem.

When my rector, Reverend Bernie Pecaro, visited me in the hospital toward the end of my stay there, he commented, "I will be very interested in watching you after you have returned to your world, Sandy, to see if you can remain 'mellowed' and not return to your old habits." I am sorry to say that some of my old habits have returned, though I try to deal with that every day. But I am improving.

The therapists cautioned me that I must be orderly and disciplined in keeping a calendar of all my scheduled appointments and allowing extra time to get there. If I allow too little time, I get nervous and anxious. If I want to stay calm, pleasant and happy, I try to allow at least 30% more time to get dressed, walk to my car, and drive to my destination. I have to allow extra time, and I must also visit the bathroom before I leave and as soon as I arrive. Stroke can impact one's bladder's "early warning system," so I must be careful. This plan never fails!

Rebecca, Nancy and my other cousins, my brothers and my friends make sure I now schedule everything and write it down. Scheduling every appointment or activity is critical for me. I do forget…a lot. They urge me (demand of me I should say) to restrict myself to two obligatory activities per day. I simply cannot attempt to try to please everyone anymore. I now am required to say "no" at least once a day. It takes a lot of vigilance to leave old (bad) habits behind, but I'm getting better at it.

Stress management has also become part of my life "A-S" (After Stroke). I had no idea what stress management was before my stroke. Now, I know. Each afternoon at 2 p.m., come what may, I must lie down and sleep for at least 15 minutes. Also, as my therapists urge, I try to schedule a 15-20 minute nap during the late morning hours. In fact, contemporary corporations are urging their top executives to do the same. Before my stroke, I *never* napped. I had that good old "Depression era" work ethic which never paid attention to the body. Work, work, work! I think I was born about 25 years too soon. It's a proven fact I am much more effective, more pleasant, and more creative when I am rested. Why am I surprised?

In the hospital, my therapists even put a yellow paper dot on my wristwatch. My instructions were that when it caught my eye, I was to stop, rest for a moment and take a deep breath. This, too, is a form of stress management. Your doctor can really help you in this regard, though it's probable that he, like most of us in America between the ages of 45 and 60, doesn't take time to do it himself.

We all have to call on our "strong" side to do more than it's supposed to do. Personally, I must make sure I don't overdo walking or carrying too much on my good side, like bags of groceries. When I carry too much in my right hand while my left arm is flaccid, my body twists and I become unbalanced. Consequently, my back, stomach and right leg muscles become overworked and sometimes cramp up because they are asked to do things they were not designed to do. Certainly I get sore. And that is discouraging, so I must avoid the habit of over-working my good right side. Most people are not aware of the constant pain stroke survivors have. It does, however, get better and better. The path to healing and solving this problem is to use our weak side as often as possible, which will help bring it back.

When the brain signals to my limbs were most confused during the early weeks after my stroke and caused my muscles to compete in opposite directions, I became spastic. I remember my cousins, Rodney and Carl, visiting me at my home after the hospital stay. Carl said, "Sandy, you are really looking better, and you seem to be better able to control your arms." Then, he and Rodney, who really love me but have terrific senses of humor, said, "Clap your hands for us." I tried, and with a clenched left hand, swung it to my right and hit my open right hand, swinging to meet it. I actually did slap them against each other.

Then, Rodney said, "Point at me with your left hand." I struggled and my left arm wobbled. I told my left forefinger to point at Rodney. But at the time, the only finger that would point straight out was my middle finger. So, I gave him "the finger." We all laughed.

Carl said, "Congratulations! We have a surprise for you. Here is an ice cream cone." He handed it to my left hand.

Spastics took over. As I tried to lick the ice cream, my left hand smashed the ice cream squarely in the middle of my forehead! We couldn't stop laughing. I think being able to laugh at myself was part of my healing.

I know that it requires my own volition, my own discipline, my own determination and effort to sustain my sense of optimism, faith and hope. I have to see the humor when it is there — even if I laugh at myself. I must persist, be resilient and tenacious, the very attributes that were part of my mental strengths before my stroke. I must remember that without question my *attitude* is my path to healing. Yet, I can't help but be grateful for the enduring love and support from those close to me who have been by my side these years. They, surely for me, have been the beacons along my path to healing.

Chapter 7

Acceptance

After a stroke you have to accept what has happened before true healing can begin. A vital step in accepting my new life was adopting a mental and spiritual state of mind that brought me past the anger, frustration and disappointment of being so crippled which affected every aspect of my life. To be sure, I was easily reminded all the time that almost in the blink of an eye, in an instant, the capabilities I did have were gone. The changes were dramatically significant and life changing. I would try to move my impacted leg or foot, my arm, my mouth, but I had to strain to do so since my brain, the computer system of the body, was "down" and sending conflicting signals to various and competing muscles all over my body. I was straining to hold my arm down with my triceps at the same time that I was straining to lift my arm with my biceps. The simplest move was such a battle that I literally exhausted myself. I had to constantly take time to rest. I had to allow my body to rebuild itself. I had to be patient, more patient than I had ever been called on to be in my entire life. I had to find hope.

There were moments when it seemed the only human response was to get mad at the world...at

God...at myself. After all, *someone* has to be blamed. But that kind of thinking is misdirected, fruitless and absurd, although it is typically human and self-destructive.

Over time, I stopped thinking that I *was* impaired and no longer who I was before my stroke. As long as I was in that anger mode, I was unhappy, depressed and good for no one. My behavior did tend to engender gestures of sympathy, which made me feel special, important, and, I'm sad to say, made me feel good. Receiving sympathy was somehow intoxicating, and I wallowed in it for weeks. I felt that I was still *a part of their world.* One so desperately needs to believe that. Being or feeling "different" separates you from others. It is terribly depressing to believe that you won't *ever* again be what you were — that your life as you knew it is *gone.* It may not have been the best life, or even a good life in some ways. But it was *your* life, and familiar, and thus "safer." It's hard to have a friend say, "You're looking better today," and adding, "We have to go," which meant, "We have to get back to our lives which you aren't part of anymore."

Constructive compassion rather than sympathy is much more beneficial. I vividly remember a dear boyhood friend, Joe Karneeb, who called me at the hospital. Joe lives in Pawtucket, Rhode Island. Our parents have been friends since long before we were born. We are the same age, and were best friends when we were seven. My family traveled to Pawtucket for the entire summer of 1945. Joe and I spent all day everyday together, playing, exploring, and bonding.

I was very surprised to hear from Joe because I hadn't seen him since we played golf together in Pawtucket a few years earlier. Now, I was in the hospital. His voice over the telephone was inspiring. "Sandy, you know we all love you and are praying for you every day. And you know we would do anything to help you bring back your healthy body. But...and you may not like hearing this, ol' buddy...it all comes down to you. You have to do it yourself. No one can do it for you. You *can* do it, Sandy. You *must* do it. We love you, Sandy." There it was — it's up to *you*, Sandy. Accept what's happened to you, and do what you have to do.

Well, to be sure, Joe was absolutely correct. My emotions were mixed. While this harsh truth was correct, I suddenly felt very lonely and separated as I heard his words. Maybe I wanted tender words of sympathy that he did not give me. My dear lifelong friend instead gave me constructive compassion, love, and a "kick in the pants." I needed his words to make me stronger, more determined, and more convinced than ever that I could do it — Joe said so! His telephone call did me more good than he could have imagined. It acknowledged and confirmed what had happened to me, and yet, it was "OK." He still loved me and welcomed me into his world. Joe's call was probably as significant to my attaining acceptance as anything else. Amazing! His "tough love" really helped me.

And that is what I am hoping this book will accomplish — that it will show that conveying compassion along with strength, confidence and love are constructive and helpful. Sympathy is fine, and, in the beginning needed, but Joe's kind of truth and honesty can convey a sense of the possible to many patients. It puts the responsibility where it must be: with the patient. In the end, even with lots of help, support and therapy treatments, "the buck stops here."

Actually, I was convinced that my new condition was so awful, so terrible, so debilitating, that for a long time I refused to even accept what had happened to me. Reaching a place of *any degree* of acceptance takes time. Lots of time. And work. And nurturing, and therapy.

As days progressed in the hospital, something began to happen to my thinking. The daily exercises, constant visits from dear friends, and limitless support from the hospital staff were beginning to bear fruit...little victories began to accumulate, to build upon one another. I kept asking questions. "Has anyone *ever* had this happen to them and then succeeded in sitting by himself and standing or walking again?" The answers from doctors and therapists also began to change from "We don't know. All strokes are different" to "Well, maybe statistically *someone* whose stroke was as serious as yours has succeeded." I was caught up in visualizing "the bell curve of statistics" where, in a class in school for example, the "curve" shows that someone got an "A," someone got an "F" and the bulk would be in the middle, forming the shape of a bell. That meant *someone had to have gotten an "A."* If this was so, then I became convinced that if *someone* with a stroke like mine, somewhere, anywhere, was able to stand or at least, if not actually walk, even "waddle," then I began to believe it was possible for me. I became determined that I would somehow, with God's help, achieve the same success. If it was possible, I began to believe that if I could visualize it, I could actualize it. If I could make standing and walking and talking and swallowing my new mental reality, I *could* achieve it. To do so, I had to become absolutely, unequivocally convinced it was possible, and absolutely unequivocally committed to achieving, no matter what it required. As I began to achieve goals, I began setting new goals. As Dr. Wayne W. Dyer, a counseling psychologist and well-known author, wrote, "You *can* have what you really, really, really, really want."

First I had to accept what had happened. Once I did, the future got better and better. There have always been setbacks, disappointments, frustrations, and constant reminders of my terrible condition. Some days, I seemed to stop progressing, other times I seemed to regress and struggle with old bad habits. And though my therapists reminded me that temporary setbacks were to be expected, I would get frustrated.

At one time, my face was totally numb on the left side, as though I had an overdose of Novocain injected in it. Even the left half of the top of my head was totally numb. I would tap the top of my bald head and actually locate a fine line down the center of the top of my head. On one side I could feel my fingernail touch my head. On the other side, I could feel nothing. I found myself checking it often, hoping…eventually accepting.

I suffered what is called "left-sided neglect," which means I lost awareness of my left side and my left visual field. The medical term is hemianopsia. I simply did not perceive the left side as existing. For example, I still sometimes ignore the left side of my face when washing. I often have to "look for" my left arm or leg when I have been sitting or lying down for a very long period of time. I just don't know where they are and tend to ignore them and not even try to use them. Accepting means, "OK, now let's deal with it."

Being literally "blind" on my entire left side and "seeing" *nothing* to my left, makes for interesting phenomena, especially at mealtimes. If the waiter places a glass of water or other beverage to the left side of my plate, I sometimes don't see it and ask them why everyone but me got a beverage. "It's right there, next to your plate," they point out. Also, I don't "see" food on the left side of my plate, so everything on the left side remains untouched. Many times, I "finish" a meal and leave all the food on the left side of the plate. It's funny in a bizarre sort of way. I may have a full plate of spaghetti, and when I am through eating, the right side is empty but the left side is still there. It is as if I had cut a straight line down the middle of the plate. When I turn my head to the left, *voila*! Wow! Where did all that food come from?

Actually, these conditions continue even now, several years after my stroke. Since my left side was, and to a lesser extent is, numb, food might linger on my left lip or cheek and I don't know it. It has gotten better, but there was a time when my left cheek was so numb, I joked that "someone pointed out that an entire leg of lamb was hanging from my left cheek." So, I learned to accept and adapt to this phenomenon. And it's helped me a lot. Today, once in a while, a rice grain may be there, but the days of a leg of lamb are over!

These conditions have been reminders of what "separated me from my old world." When I asked, "What has happened to me?" the answer would be something like "your brain has been attacked" or "your brain has been insulted" or "your brain has been badly injured. We don't know why or what caused it. But it was severe." When I considered asking the question "why me?" I always knew the obvious answer was "why not you?" So, I never asked that question.

Now, when I speak to groups, I sometimes say, "Nearly half of my brain was destroyed. And now, I have a valid reason for being a 'half-wit'."

All during the Pinecrest rehabilitation period, there were always reasons for frustration and anger. How can I stand if I don't know where my left leg is? If I can't stand, how can I walk? If I can't put my left foot under me, how can I stand? If I try to move my leg forward and my brain turns on the counter muscles simultaneously, how am I going to ever move my leg? If I get exhausted simply trying to grip a doorknob with my left hand and my muscles are pulling against each other, how am I ever going to get around? I can't even propel myself with a wheelchair.

Rebecca and her assistants, the young men, who pushed my wheelchair or helped move me about, were so encouraging that I slowly began the process of envisioning what I *could* do more than what I *could not* do. I began to view my life from a half-full glass perspective than a half-empty glass. But what a slow process it was. It took hours, days, weeks and months, one day at a time. I had to take on the attitude of "another day of therapy, another day toward independence." I began to *believe*. But, I couldn't begin until I learned to accept my fate. I slowly emerged from the swamp-like place of "will this horrible movie ever end" to a place of "I can get past this." As I write, I am reminded that my loving family was going through the same struggles I was enduring. But they didn't have the benefit of having the reassurance of the therapists each day, encouraging, nurturing. So, it was very hard for them. All loving caregivers suffer along with the stroke survivor...each and every day. We mustn't forget that.

Some people say, "God never gives you more than you can handle" and maybe that is so. But I was aware that if that is true, then God took me right to the edge of my limitations. I remember telling my brother Ernie during an early visit, "This is the worst, most painful, time of my life. If all the horrible, painful times in my life were combined, and then multiplied by a thousand times, this would still be the worst." And then I told him, remembering what we went through during my mother's terminal illness only a year before, "If the doctors ask you for permission to put me on life support machines to keep me living like this, let me go. I don't want to live if it's going to be like this. If I must, I'm ready to go, Ernie."

I asked God to teach me patience. "God," I said, "I want patience and I want it now!" He must have smiled lovingly and thought, "My son, be careful what you ask for...you may just get it...especially when you ask for patience." Learning patience, especially for a chronically impatient person, is very, very hard.

I recognized the best way for me to rid myself of the anger that I held inside for months after my stroke was to forgive those whom I felt had really treated me badly and, in my opinion, had taken unreasonable and unnecessary actions that injured me so much.

Bible study helped me learn how to forgive. By forgiving these few individuals I was released from that debilitating, painful anger.

As I sometimes tell my friends who are honestly surprised at my progress, who know how terrible it has been, "I am a miracle in progress." I truly feel God has healed me, and while my calendar may seem quicker than His, I am the recipient of His miracle.

I am a "believer" and am convinced there are angels who message for God and that there are such things as miracles. I believe with all my being that God has healed me in so many ways, and that He is not done with me yet...that I have more to do with my life. To paraphrase Dr. Wayne Dyer, who speaks the truth so eloquently, "I must not leave this earth without having sung my song." Watching Dr. Dyer speak, and reading his books is always an enriching experience for me. He reminds me in his special televised presentations and his books that from the "falls" we experience in life, and surely a catastrophic stroke qualifies as a "fall," we are given the opportunities to attain higher levels of

Life. Listening to this admonition he attributes to the kabala, I realize I must use this stroke to propel myself to a higher purpose, a higher understanding, and a place from which I will fulfill my destiny. And, by doing this, I open myself to God's power, God's will, and turn control of my life over to Him, allowing Him to come to my aid. Whether one believes in God or calls Him the universe, the essence of this is a person's *relationship* with God, or the universe. Within each of us is that power to literally change ourselves. I had to create a whole new reality, a new vision for my life. It had to come from within to be sure, but I was convinced that I could do it alone. Now, I am convinced that I had to call on my God, my Friend. I had to *know* what I wanted, what I *intended* (Dr. Dyer's word), and do so with passion. I believe I *invited* the power of God, the universe, if you will, to come to my aid. I want to enjoy my new life as much as I can. I accept what has happened and want to live my life to the fullest, come what may. Life is too precious to squander, to waste. There is no benefit to anger, depression or self-pity. We must *accept* life as a gift and *live it*!

Chapter 8

Picking Up The Pieces

It's all about building new relationships

I have found true treasures in the friendships I had before my stroke, both male and female, and I have found extraordinary joy in new friendships. Those I treasured most were with the kindest, most caring, most giving and most optimistic friends. I have drawn on their strength and sincere love for me. My family and friends were enormous sources of comfort and strength. I am convinced every survivor must learn to *accept* gifts of kindness and draw on our strengths, no matter how angry and depressed we feel. These feelings of anger and depression have to be overcome. And visitors want very much to help. Let them. They can provide a path that counters the natural feelings of "despair, separateness, aloneness and loneliness" that are to be expected and dealt with.

Every time loving friends or relatives visited me early on in the hospital, I wanted to touch their hand or their face. I tried hard to smile, even with the severe headaches and hiccups.

Family and friends were worried, wonderful, affectionate and patient with me. Like anyone paralyzed, physically and emotionally, like most stroke victims, I felt "less" than I was, and in many ways helpless. I felt I was not the person they knew before. Unfairly, and I think this is true of most of us, I did not give them credit for believing in me, or wanting to give so much to *me*. Here I was, not believing in them.

I am fortunate to have had many loving family members and friends who were by my side when I most needed them. There is a great, almost overwhelming feeling of being a "victim." It seems we want to crawl into a fetal position and sleep our lives away, without anyone watching us. There are moments we experience that are similar to other post-tragedy experiences; like a sudden awareness of the impacts of divorce, or when the "death" of a former life takes place and we want to be alone in our emotional suffering. These feelings are to be expected. They are normal and typical. But we must learn that *we are not alone*. There is help and support all around us in these times of need. Caregivers should expect this terrible period of sadness and apathy. Anger and impatience can be children of these feelings, so, sometimes, it can be as difficult, if not more so, for the loving, but worried friend or spouse. That's when we need our friends the most.

There are people available through the hospital services, religious, private or public agencies who want to, and will and do provide emotional support. My urging is that one must reach out to find those people. Most hospitals or rehabilitation clinics have support groups of stroke survivors who discuss together solutions and concerns to nearly every problem. In many cases, simply asking for help begins the healing process by confronting the fact that you have a need. And by confronting that need and seeking assistance, we are, in truth, reflecting a sense of optimism that life will be better with that assistance. Reaching out and asking for help is the start of rebuilding relationships in a different way. It is particularly true if the survivor actively seeks out to a receptive, supportive friend or relative.

Even though I was lucky to have had so many friends and family visit, there were times in the hospital, and later at home, when I wanted to reconnect and rebuild those relationships beyond their visitations. I found that one of my best and most "friendly" way of reaching out was taking in hand the telephone, conveniently attached to my bed rail. I happen to be very adept at the telephone and enjoy talking a lot (as my friends will attest).

By using the telephone, I knew the other person on the other end of the line could not see me. That in itself was a bit comforting, because I was lying in my bed, unable to move my body, or use my left arm and hand. Fortunately, my speech was impaired only for a few months, having had most of the damage in the right side of my brain, but having right side damage also made me impulsive.

There were times of loneliness and a need to talk to a friend or family member, or even an acquaintance thousands of miles away, when I would impulsively pick up the phone and call. Sometimes, since it might happen late at night, I recommend you get a prior "OK." There are times when someone simply doesn't want a phone call. It could become a real test of that friendship. That call may be something the stroke victim might need, but a sleeping friend has receiving a late night call a very low priority! Timing is always important.

The telephone became a good means of communication for me during my hospital stay and long after when I would call from my own bed at home. I began to call dear friends, and even friends of friends,

who were local or even out of state. If it was late on the
East Coast, I would dial someone in a later time zone,
like in Logan, Utah, or Los Angeles, California. I got a
lot of comfort from carefully selected friends who
would receive my nocturnal calls after midnight my
time, but only nine o'clock their time. So, aside from
the impact on my phone bill, I found it was easy for me
to speak to those who could not see me in my
paralyzed, helpless condition, and treated me as an
"equal." Over time, as my speech improved, they
would compliment me on my progress. Those
comments were very helpful in improving my attitude.
Each call I made seemed to bring me added strength,
optimism and encouragement to continue my battle. We
would talk about *everything*, and sometimes talk for
more than an hour. It was, after all, "my dime." (Dime?
How old am I?)

Everyone, especially those who have suffered a
severe tragedy or even aging, needs social contact.
Many survivors who have relatives (presumed to be
loving, caring and worried) near enough to visit must
find a way to take it upon themselves to "reach out."
Sometimes, depending on the person, it can be better to
visit over the telephone, since the "visitor" cannot see
the caller or witness the incapacity of the stroke
survivor, or, perhaps, physically cannot visit. It's also
more convenient than actually getting dressed, driving
or riding to see you. That phone call can be very
comforting. Today, it is even better and easier than it
was in 1994, the year of my early convalescence.
Today, one can simply pick up the handle, or better yet,
punch the speaker button on the phone and tap the
redial button. It's so easy.

Now, as my mobility has improved, "e-mail" is
for me. I must type with only my right hand, but I'm
learning now to use a voice-activated e-mail and letter

typing program. But the telephone is still my favorite since I prefer the sound of someone's voice. And now, the cost of long distance and even local calls is much lower, seemingly getting cheaper each day. Isn't competition wonderful? Maybe one day the government will even lower their telephone taxes...? which currently constitute a major portion of my phone bill... then my bill will come down. Probably not. After all, the government doesn't have any competition...yet.

But I digress.

"Reaching out" by telephone or otherwise by the stroke survivor, or even the harried and overburdened spouse/caregiver, is a great means of coping with moments of feelings of despair or "aloneness." Societal and personal connections, as well as relationship rebuilding are vital parts of the healing process.

As I have been asked more frequently to speak before stroke support groups, and to visit survivors as "one who has been there," I have learned that those who are dealing with "post-stroke-syndrome" depression, anger, apathy and sadness, are those who are not even alone at home a large part of the time. Even if a survivor has a spouse or caregiver at home, it is important to the healing process to interact with others outside the home or the immediate family. Meeting with support groups or even small groups of friends or acquaintances can be excellent, uplifting experiences. Activities with others of similar interests are preferred over activities done alone. For example, I finally overcame a strong reluctance to attend acrylic and oil painting classes at 10 a.m. each Saturday morning. While painting is done by one's self, the social interaction in the classes was really excellent and became a powerful inducement to my healing. I truly enjoyed the friendships I gained with my wonderful teacher, Nancy, and the other students whose ages ranged from youngsters (8-10) to elders up to 80 years old. Everyone was focused on learning to paint. They weren't focused on me or the woman who had a hip problem, but were so friendly, kind, and helpful to both of us (especially if I inadvertently knocked over my wet painting, kicked their easel leg with my "brainless" left foot, or spilled my cup filled with colored water and brushes). I found that painters are basically patient, understanding people.

Picking up the pieces of one's life is better accomplished by rebuilding prior relationships. I have devoted a great deal of my emotions and time to reconnecting with people I haven't seen or been with in years, sometimes more than forty years. There is what I would call a "patina" that accompanies those old friendships. Sometimes we visit in person, or more frequently — weekly — sometimes on the telephone, and now, by e-mail. I exchange messages with acquaintances from my college years and from high school. Warm memories quickly recall, for both parties, happier, innocent days of our youth. I have found great cheer, joy, and abundant good feelings, together with amazingly encouraging sensations, from friends who remember our good times.

I have found other avenues to be helpful, too. The other source of new friendships is participating with new groups of people. One cannot be afraid of meeting new people, making new connections, and establishing new, and sometimes better, friendships.

There may be pre-stroke relationships that we might choose not to rebuild, or with some we choose *not* to pick up the pieces. Those that would not bring good feelings of joy or happiness are better avoided. People who brought pain prior to the stroke will likely bring pain *after* the stroke. Thankfully, those people didn't visit or contact me, and I had the good sense not to contact them. Those people with whom we might not have had so great relationships are better left "sleeping." My advice is to leave them alone.

After I left Pinecrest Rehabilitation Hospital, I continued several therapies on an outpatient basis for nearly a year. During that time, I learned to drive again, first on the parking lot of a nearby shopping center after hours (so I wouldn't hit someone) and then on local streets — I finally graduated to Interstate 95, a really unfriendly place for the uncertain novice driver. I was filled with a renewed sense of freedom. I began to feel I could now reconnect with people because now I could drive to them rather than always be picked up in my wheelchair or with my cane.

Before my stroke, I had enjoyed having dinner or simply visiting together with Jan, who had become my guardian angel in the hospital. After I could drive again, I called her. "Dinner?" I asked.

"I'd love to, Sandy."

My self-confidence grew. "Saturday at six?"

"You are on," she laughed.

And so began a resumption of sorts for this 56-year-old single man.

We had a wonderful evening at a fine restaurant and talked all evening. I felt like I was on a cloud. After all, Jan was a beautiful, delightful woman any man would have been proud to accompany. I felt secure in Jan's company because Jan had been with me during my lowest periods. She was kind, caring, and sweet to me. She made me feel so good. My confidence and self-image went from negative to positive overnight. Because of her, I knew I had no reason to be anywhere near anyone who did not make me feel good about myself. I really didn't have the emotional reserves to deal with them anyway. Jan and I formed a fond relationship filled with respect. We are still good friends.

I began to venture out more. I developed a loving, even romantic, relationship with a woman. It has taken me nearly six years, with some false starts, because there were times when I was so emotionally vulnerable that I would get scared and pull back, preferring a "best friend" relationship. It became "safer" for both parties. Now I relate better, am more likely to share my feelings, and am more sensitive, more creative and more loving. Some have said that my stroke brought out my "feminine side." That's OK with me. It feels good.

Picking up the pieces of one's life after a severe stroke requires wanting to and taking the initiative to help make it happen. An old saying I like certainly holds true for stroke survivors:

Some people make things happen,
Some people watch things happen
Some people wonder what happened.

We all wonder what happened. But the way to healing and coping with this terrible tragedy is to commit to picking up the pieces of our lives and finding ways to live, really live again. It means making the effort, surrounding yourself with friends and those who bring you hope, laughter, encouragement, and a will to live in their lives again. You can do it if you try.

Chapter 9

Teaching As A Human Being

Let your light so shine before others,
that they may see your good works,
and glorify your Father who is in heaven.
Matthew 5:16

By overcoming tragedy and simply "being," we become teachers. Sometimes, the simplest advice or counsel as a human being is the most effective and most remembered.

One of my mentors was the father of a dear friend of mine. He was enjoying his 95th birthday. I asked, "Mr. Maloof, after all these years of living a good life, what advice would you give me?" I don't recall what I expected him to say at the time, but I was pleasantly surprised when he responded by putting his hand gently on my shoulder, and after a pause looking into my eyes, and, almost in a whisper, answered, "Sandy, don't worry." Imagine, 95 years of living came to "*don't worry.*" I've never forgotten that, but still find myself foolishly worrying about something. Not worrying is not easy for me. But it happens less and less. Here was a man who had emigrated from northern

Lebanon as a poor, young boy, settled in a very small town named Copper Hill, Tennessee, eventually owned a dry goods store, raised a loving family, and invested well. He was always surrounded by his wife, children, grandchildren, great-grandchildren, and friends. He was blessed to have them with him when he died at the age of 100. All those who knew and thus loved him cherish his memory. *"Don't worry..."*

Now I'm a "teacher," and I have come to realize since my stroke, my teaching is best exemplified by *overcoming adversity and living each day as fully and as happily as possible.* To do that with grace and wisdom requires becoming more a human being and less a human doing. I believe, since this life is all about learning, it means overcoming obstacles and growing closer to God. My struggles as a result of my stroke have better prepared me for this task of teaching. I certainly look on life differently and, since teaching can be, to a large extent, simply setting an example, I am now a better and more effective teacher than I was before my stroke. More and more, I am "being," and less and less "doing." Although, I must confess, while the experience has been a difficult life-changing one, an epiphany, my proclivity toward involvement and the compulsive behavior of a "human doing" have not altogether disappeared. I still take on more than I should and each year I resolve "to do better next year." It's a constant effort to continue to adjust to my new realities, and it's an experience I am trying to learn to savor and enjoy. I'm learning to say to myself, "Stop and smell the roses," and really understand what that means.

I find myself more eager to help others. I frequently give talks to civic and support groups. Before my stroke I spoke on global politics, local politics, and taught real estate economics at a college in

Georgia. All those subjects have been and remain of great interest to me, yet are no longer part of my favored subjects. Now, I advocate preservation of the environment, of natural open space, of living in better relationships with my neighbors. I use more of my time and efforts seeking support and grants for children's and other health groups. I am a participant more than a leader. I spend more time at church and with my friends, and am more apt to spend time in meditation. Less time is spent being busy and "doing," and more time is spent listening, observing, thinking and "being." And others tell me they are learning more from me simply by watching, witnessing. I think this is true of anyone who has overcome a terrible human tragedy. And that gives added meaning to our struggle.

The experience of my stroke virtually jerked me onto a different path, onto one of concern for other individuals' needs, of a healthy sense of giving to others. I came to a more spiritual, peaceful world of person-to-person relationships, of being *with* God and carrying out His work, not mine, with individuals. In short, I have become a "human being," more sensitive to the world. As a writer and an artist, I have made friends with other artists and would-be artists, and with budding and successful writers — people who love, create and give of themselves, instead of those I was involved with or battled in my stressful life before my stroke — bankers, businessmen, politicians, and government bureaucrats. My interest in, and awareness, of colors, of wildlife, of nature, even of colors in cloud formations has grown. I became totally aware of the morning sunrises, rainbows, flowers, and trees. By writing, I find myself more thoughtful, less anxious, less competitive, and happy to interact with so many people on a friendly one-on-one basis. As this happens, I forget that I ever had a stroke. And as I behave this way, many people are surprised to learn or forget I ever suffered a severe cerebral hemorrhage.

It has been a revelation to "be there" as these changes have taken place within me. I seek to share my experiences and new awareness with others. Certainly, like everyone I've ever known, it *never* occurred to me that I would *ever, ever* suffer a catastrophic stroke or other life-changing injury. We delude ourselves that "it always happens to someone else."

A good example of what I am describing about my new life and teaching as a human being took place during one of my therapy sessions at the local therapy clinic. I was asked by the therapist assistant to speak to a recent stroke survivor whose name was Seymour. I had met Seymour earlier during group therapy sessions at Pinecrest Rehabilitation Hospital and watched him struggle through his therapeutic regimen. His body would twist and his left foot and knee would lurch at each step. The effort was hard for him and threw him off balance; consequently, he would get very tired after only a few steps. It was difficult for all of us, but more difficult for Seymour, a lovable, but very sad man. He was about 80 years old, small of stature, and bewildered by this catastrophe that had befallen him. He was depressed and terribly alone emotionally.

When I went to his cubicle, I found him lying on the cot on his side. I asked, "How are you feeling, Seymour?"

He looked up at me and I watched as tears welled-up in his eyes and overflowed onto his cheeks. "Sandy, I want to die," he murmured. "I can't do this anymore."

I felt helpless, but gathered all the strength and positiveness I could muster.

I was new at this sort of thing, and searched my mind for a connection or a hook of a comment that would help me to gain his confidence.

"You told me you have four grandchildren, Seymour. Tell me their names." I felt, if anything, Seymour's love for his grandchildren would be my best opportunity. We had spoken a few weeks earlier about his love for his family.

"They're beautiful children," he whispered.

"Can you sit up and visit with me, Seymour?"

"I can tell you about my grandchildren."

"What are their names?" I asked.

"Joel is eight, Sarah is six, Max is four, and 'little Seymour', the baby, is two. They are so beautiful." As he eagerly repeated their names and ages to me, I am sure I saw the beginnings of a proud smile in the corner of his lips.

"Well, Seymour, don't they love you?"

"Of course they love me. A lot, maybe as much as I love them."

"Well, my dear friend, if you die, they won't be able to come to see you, hug you and sit on your lap. And they *want* to hug you and sit on your lap. You can't deprive them of that, Seymour. Can you?"

His chin dropped and he looked down.

"Seymour, I believe you told me you served in Europe during World War II. Isn't that true?"

He nodded his head and looked up at me.

I looked into his eyes. "I know you were in some dangerous spots in Europe and faced death, didn't you? And wasn't that frightening?" I asked. "Wasn't that worse than now? And you mustered all your resolve then and came out alright, didn't you?"

"Yes," he replied. And he began to remember.

"Seymour, let's pray together."

"Okay."

And we prayed. I reminded myself that my friend was of the Jewish faith and I respected that; thus, I chose my words carefully and with sensitivity. I spoke, asking God to hear us, and thanking Him for all our blessings. I asked God to forgive us our sins and to bring to Seymour strength, peace, and understanding.

I placed my hand on Seymour's head; then, Seymour put his hand on my knee where I sat next to him. I asked God to give Seymour the courage and patience to endure this terrible experience, to bring His love to Seymour, his wife, children, and grandchildren. I also prayed to God to heal Seymour and me, to give us faith.

He looked at me with tears welling up, believing his healing was already taking place. I think we really bonded that day and he was better able to cope from then on. It was a difficult, and yet wonderful, emotional moment for both of us, secluded behind the drawn curtain of his cubicle.

When I was finished, I kissed Seymour on his forehead, hugged him, and told him I loved him and that God loved him. As I got up, I held Seymour's hand. He looked at me and said, "Sandy, you've improved so much. Do you think I can too?"

"Yes, Seymour, I believe you can too."

"Thank you, Sandy. Please visit me again."

As I pulled the curtain back and stepped out of Seymour's cubicle, my friend Sol, in his cubicle across from Seymour's, pulled his curtain open and looked at me. I had tears in my eyes.

"Will you pray with me, Sandy?"

"Of course I'll pray with you, Sol."

"Are you a Catholic priest?" he asked.

"No, Sol, I'm not a Catholic priest. I'm an Episcopalian, and I believe God loves all of us. I give thanks to Him every day and ask for strength and healing."

"Please pray for me now," he asked.

"Of course," I replied. And I did, and when I had, Sol, my good friend and fellow traveler, clasped my hand. He looked at me so peacefully and whispered, "Thank you."

This emotional experience was very rewarding to me. Since my stroke and intensive rehabilitation, I want to help anyone less fortunate than I am who need a hand. In this way, I am an example to them, convincing them that they are not alone, and that the future can be brighter. I speak before groups of seniors all the time. Sometimes, it seems just appearing before them, after they are told of my near-death cerebral hemorrhage, reinforces an awareness of the lessons of determination and faith we all have experienced, perhaps long ago. I feel a deep sense of harmony now, a wonderful feeling of fulfillment and grace. This stroke gave me the opportunity to see my life from a totally different perspective. I can now see that I can enjoy life in very different ways. It is my hope that others who have suffered a stroke can also see that their lives can be enriched in new ways. With a positive attitude, one can find a rewarding form of happiness. One can teach by example and live a fulfilling and enjoyable life. This is how one can turn a devastating brain attack called a stroke into one's personal *Stroke of Genius*.

By showing I have overcome this terrible stroke and have returned to an active, yet mellower, life, I am told often that I am an inspiration "all over town." People look on me as an example of success in overcoming a horrible catastrophe of a crushing blow to my health and my life. I am told that they appreciate more who I am now instead of what I accomplished in my career. And that makes me very happy. It seems that I am teaching simply by "being," not by "doing," and that is why I am sharing these feelings and experiences in this book. You, my dear reader, will be the best judge of my success.

Chapter 10

The Therapeutic Odyssey Continues

Cruise Control

Life, it is correctly said, is a journey. It is a continuum, a process. For stroke survivors, it is even more so. We have to understand that we must focus on training our injured brains to learn more a different way, to somehow adapt to our injury. We must take on unfamiliar therapeutic activities and conditioning as part of our lifestyle. We need to find ways to enable ourselves to become, once again, socially and physically active and involved. We can and must turn away from atrophy, apathy, despair, and sheer boredom. We can and should also seek alternatives that are adventurous, pleasurable, productive and inspiring. I found various disciplines to be very helpful. Even though, in some cases, their availability may vary, I suggest the following forms of therapy, and I encourage stroke survivors to seek them out and try them.

Weight bearing can be done at one's home and has been the most helpful therapy in restoring my left arm capabilities. Returning my left arm usage has been a much slower process and has taken much longer than with my left leg. If we do not use our weak limbs as often as possible, we continue to ignore their very existence, which only exacerbates the loss of capabilities. Using the leg to stand, walk, or even placing it on the floor while sitting, are forms of weight bearing. One is doing this almost all the time except when lying down, of course. Weight bearing exercises for the arm require using the left arm (and maybe with assistance from the right hand) to bear weight by being on all fours on the floor and/or doing push-ups against the wall or countertops or exercising with light weights. This improves circulation and range of motion. I remember asking Rebecca recently (fully knowing the answer) if it would help "bring control back to my left arm sooner if I got on all fours and did push-ups 30 or 40 times a day." She smiled and replied, "Of course all that would help. The more you can weight bear, the faster better control will return. *And it will return!*" Recent research programs have indicated significant neuro-tissue response when the therapeutic usage of weight bearing on one's weak-side is concentrated and intensive.

Hyperbaric therapy is an innovative treatment I was told about one year after my stroke. It has long been successfully utilized in helping burn victims or diabetics in their healing process. It necessitated my driving one hour to a clinic in Ft. Lauderdale. That was the only regional private clinic that I could locate that was well-recommended. A local hospital had the equipment and capability, but in late 1994, it was used primarily for burn patients or scuba divers who had gotten the bends. I was told that this high-pressure oxygen treatment might accelerate the healing of my brain cells. My insurance company did not yet approve the treatment, so I paid for it myself. The weekly one-hour sessions for a couple of months seemed to help my restoration. Brain scans clearly showed improvement.

Today, hyperbaric therapy has become recognized by many insurance companies as a bona fide stroke therapy and, as a result, it is often covered. Now, it is much more readily available. Try it. It really can, in many cases, help restore injured brain cells.

Dolphin therapy, working with dolphins, is another remarkable experience. Dolphins are so intelligent and so compatible with humans that their very nearness is a powerful inducement for therapeutic patients to try much harder to stretch their capabilities. I went from kneeling on all fours in my living room to weight bearing on a floating deck with a dolphin swimming around me. Touching that lovable, large, smooth-skinned, smiling, intelligent dolphin was an irresistible enticement and forced me to *emphatically* weight bear on my left arm and stretch far beyond where I would normally reach to expand my range of motion. Just to touch the dolphin, as it knowingly swam by, was exhilarating. How that dolphin knew to circle and swim so slowly past me, just a few inches farther away from me than the previous pass, and then return to my out-stretched hand was amazing. But it worked! As I observed young, handicapped patients touching or riding the dolphins at Dr. David Nathanson's beautiful, lagoon-like clinic on Key Largo in the Florida Keys, I became convinced that the reward of touching a dolphin, being *in* the water *with* the dolphins, and, for children, being in the arms of the therapist near a dolphin, is compelling. It *demands* a response from the patient. Children, especially, respond beyond normal "mainstream" therapies and seem to improve dramatically right before your eyes. Dr. Nathanson has had such great success with his dolphin therapy, carried out by his expert and dedicated licensed therapists, that he has a constant waiting list of patients from all over the world. The use of dolphins in treating patients with a variety of neurological deficits has been, and is noted, in many success stories. These treatments successfully encourage a shift from apathy, resignation, lethargy or indifference to excitement and a noticeably increased desire for therapy sessions, especially with children.

Hippotherapy, riding on horseback (hippo is Greek for horse), is an excellent form of therapy that I have undertaken over the past few years with Rebecca's encouragement, guidance and supervision. Research has found that the rhythm and movement of a horse is so similar to that of human beings that it really stimulates brain retraining of the relationships of body parts. It "reminds" the mind where the left hip is when the right hip is somewhere else (up, down, forward, back…). I attribute a good deal of my improvement in my walking coordination to hippotherapy. It has produced near-miracles for many patients, especially those with autism, cerebral palsy, brain injury, and the like. It is enriching to be around these children, watching how happy they become as they too share beautiful moments sitting on a horse in a farm-like setting, wearing their helmets, and riding safely as the horse slowly walks within the riding ring with its whitewashed boards under blue skies out among nature. Rebecca arranged for me to have hippotherapy treatments weekly at a horse farm for nearly a year. For another series of sessions, we relocated to Horses for the Handicapped, a remarkable nationwide program.

Hippotherapy has really helped me in using my left side trunk muscles and training my hip movement to enable me to walk smoother and consume a lot less energy. The benefits to my left arm movement have been mainly directed to reducing the tone of my muscles. I have found that after hippotherapy sessions, my left arm has less spasticity and responds better.

Recreational therapy was first introduced to me during my second month in Pinecrest Rehabilitation Hospital. At first, the class started with very simple and rudimentary tasks. There were about six adults who, with the guidance of our recreational therapist, were offered various options of crafts and painting. We could weave simple patterns, paint with watercolors, finger-paint, draw, and at the same time, have fun with other patients. It helped us laugh, enjoy and be socially active beyond our daily hours of other therapeutic regimens. It was helpful to all of us to become a "social animals" again.

Other recreational activities that were fun and "adventurous" included going to the supermarket or the park. It was a bridge for us from the solitary existence of our hospital rooms, the therapy gym, and the sessions in the small cubicle offices of the speech therapist or psychotherapist. Recreational therapy, though apparently not considered a high priority in improving one's physical capabilities, is, I have found, very important in rebuilding one's emotional healing, awareness of the world and one's place in it. By actively participating in these recreational activities, rebuilding camaraderie and becoming socially active, one's sense of esteem, confidence level, improved social capabilities, and a growing feeling of joy can actually substantially improve one's physical rebuilding and healing. Painting became a wonderful activity for me. I joined classes and quickly looked forward to each weekly session in spite of my impairments.

Nancy Cunningham, my art teacher and gallery owner, urged me to improve, paint, improve and paint. I had to sit at a table during my painting classes because I couldn't stand long or hold a pallet in my left hand. I chose to paint in water-soluble acrylics, instead of oils, which are far more difficult to use, especially when cleaning the brushes. As it turned out, I often knocked over the cup of water on my table with my left hand as I stood up. Imagine how messy oils and turpentine would have been and how much help I would have needed to clean up. It was bad enough with acrylic-colored water spilled everywhere. But then it would get worse, just as Murphy's Law states: "If it can get worse, it will." And it did.

Sometimes, when I would stand up to step back from the canvas on the easel so I could get a longer perspective, my "tag-a-long" neglected left hand would drag across my pallet gathering various colors of paint. Ohhh! Oops! Damn! Spill. The water cup would be clobbered too! Now what to do? My left hand was literally covered in great globs of reds, yellows, white, blue and variations in between. As I was clumsily limping to get away the first time it happened, I was embarrassed and surprised at what I saw and tipped over the leg of my easel, tossing my 30 x 40 inch canvas onto someone else's pallet.

The next few times it happened, I decided to use my paint-covered left hand and plopped and rubbed it across a clean canvas.

It came out beautifully, but very "modern." I was offered more for that accidental painting than I was offered for my meticulously detailed seascape.

So much for the tastes of my public.

In time, Nancy encouraged me to host, with her, an evening exhibit. So, I invited family members and friends, presented hors d'oeuvres, and held a very successful one-man showing. What a thrill! I couldn't believe it. Six paintings were purchased that first evening. What a boost to my self-confidence! I was ecstatic. I even wore a beret. This experience proved to me I was surely returning to the world — not as a real estate executive or civic activist or businessman.

Rather, I was returning as another kind of person in keeping with the emotional and physical changes that occur to some people after a severe brain injury. I was becoming perceived as an unassuming artist and writer.

After several years of reluctance to venture near a golf course, I finally agreed to join in another form of recreational therapy. I grew to love it, and attended the sessions weekly. The Palm Beach County Parks Department and St. Mary's Hospital recreational therapists offered group golf lessons for the impaired at the Okeeheelee Golf Course in West Palm Beach. At first, I didn't want to go near a golf course or even try to play golf again, thinking I would be clumsy, inept, delay my friends, and stumble everywhere. I formed all sorts of excuses — like I wouldn't be able to swing without falling down...I have no balance...I couldn't walk up the slopes to the green...I couldn't walk in or out of the sand traps...and, I would get too tired. I put so many obstacles in my thought process that I just put the idea of even playing golf again out of my mind.

I am so glad Joanie, the recreational therapist at St. Mary's Hospital, never gave up on me and urged me to participate in the program. About a dozen of us, recovering from a variety of illnesses including stroke, Guillain-Barre syndrome, spinal injuries, brain injuries and Parkinson's were invited to sign up for a series of four Saturday morning lessons.

We all helped one another, supported one another, visited over coffee and donuts, and received abundant praise and instruction from Donna White, our wonderful PGA golf professional, and our recreational therapists. While I struggled swinging with just my right arm, Lyman, who became a good friend of mine, had a difficult time gripping the club handle as a result of his bout with Guillain-Barre syndrome. Donna helped us overcome our individual handicaps. For instance, at first, she had to tape Lyman's hands to the club handle. We all learned to laugh at our mishaps and cheered one another when we did something right. There was camaraderie each of us enjoyed. Donna was so patient with each of us as she and the young and enthusiastic therapists and aides, Joanie, Fiona, Briana and Jackie, helped us and cheered us on. All of our exercises, while dedicated to building self-esteem, improving our balance and weight shifting, improved our abilities to socially interact. At the same time, we were taught to play a little golf under our new circumstances. And we were relearning to enjoy life and rejoin the world.

I found myself marveling at the determination, sense of adventure and sense of peace my colleagues exhibited. Several rode in special electric carts. When it was time to hit their golf balls, they would lock their carts in place, spin their seats to the side, and with a somewhat miniaturized club about three feet long, take a swing and actually hit the ball 50 or 60 yards. To watch the wide smile of joy after succeeding was worth every effort exerted! What an uplifting experience and sense of accomplishment.

I can't believe how well I relearned to hit the ball. I am now hitting the wedge up to 60 yards, the eight iron up to 100 yards and, for the real stretch, the five wood or 4 iron, my favorite, 150 yards — straight, too, all using only my right arm! I can do it! I *can* play golf again! And, I am glad to say, following Donna's instructions on weight shift, body position and arm movements made most of my shots straight, even though my left side is not pulling or moving correctly. I still have a way to go. Sometimes, though I am able to hit the ball well on the fairways, I might not concentrate on the greens and putt the ball 130 feet.

Without question, our self-esteem is improved too when we get a chance to watch a healthy "weekend duffer" at the driving range watching him slice, top or hook the ball once in a while and we might out-drive him! Having a sense of humor can be a great salvation no matter where you are or what you are doing. I am having a wonderful time now that I can hit a golf ball without falling down! (It's so hard to get up that I'm *really* glad I don't do that anymore.) But then, the next lesson was hitting from the sand traps. Uh-oohhh!

By participating in this wonderful experience, I have come to realize that I love getting outdoors back on the putting green, the driving range and out in the open spaces. Now I even look forward to getting on the golf course and playing a few of holes of golf.

I have become a believer in recreational therapy and its importance in our lives. I am indebted to Donna and her charges for the enthusiasm and energy that have become part of our lives. I agree with the recreational therapists in their belief that the patient's leisure interests *must* be integrated into the therapy process so one can resume a pre-stroke lifestyle of activities among the rest of the world. I even wrote the County Commission a laudatory letter complimenting them, The Parks and Recreation Department, and Donna, for what they were doing for us "impaired" citizens.

As I have progressed, mostly after my first year following the stroke, I began seeking additional convenient means of reconditioning my body. Much of it was directed toward expanding the range of motion of my left arm and hand, which, happily, were becoming more mobile and responsive. So, I began taking the advice of many people, including therapists and my physiatrist (a doctor who specializes in post-stroke rehabilitation therapy). They urged me to "get into the swimming pool and exercise." I began aqua therapy.

The exercises included walking across the pool in waist-deep water to rebuild my leg strength, help me improve my balance and increase my sense of confidence. In deeper water, I rotated my left arm against the water. Working against the water while exercising my arms and legs really works! It not only increased my range of motion...overhead swings, lateral moves up and down, but also allowed me to perform strokes as though I were swimming again. Everyone urges aqua therapy for good reasons.

Physical conditioning therapy became important to me as my new life has evolved, even six years after my stroke, and I expect it to continue for years to come. As I began replacing my business and civic activities with painting lessons, writing, and continued physical therapy, I still needed to devote myself to protecting my body and attitude from the aging process as well. I found that I needed to somehow, under the circumstances, strengthen my body, increase my stamina and rebuild my endurance capabilities in order to live a higher quality of life.

I was very much aware that I couldn't walk for long without getting tired and even exhausted. I was napping often and becoming very sedentary. Others who have suffered a stroke find themselves wheelchair-bound or spend much of their lives in their bed or on the couch watching too much television. Reading is difficult, tiring, and not enjoyable for many of us. Using one hand, possible eyesight difficulties or attention span deficiencies, to say nothing of the constant pain, physical inability to move around, and much less mobility, also contributes to the sedentary lifestyle. But we must find a way to recondition our bodies, restore our stamina, get active again, meet new people, and energize ourselves.

After a few years, I became convinced I seriously needed to begin conditioning therapy. I considered joining a gym and rebuilding my left side. Clearly, my left arm and leg were very much weaker and smaller than my right arm and leg. Of course, I depended on my right leg to stand up and sit down. When I walked, I noticed the muscle tone in my left limbs had really deteriorated, atrophied and was not improving discernibly. Yet, like most people over 50, the idea of going to the gym was terribly intimidating. All the television ads featured incredibly *muscular* men *and* women. They had gorgeous, curvaceous bodies that would make me look like the "infamous 97 pound weakling."

I really had to overcome a huge psychological obstacle to put myself in the midst of these beautiful people in their colorful, skintight leotards. My limbs were small to begin with, and now, I had really small limbs on my left side, and walked with a limp with my left hand near my crotch. I was nearing 60 years old, had lots of gray hair (and exposed scalp), and, if I allowed myself to think about it, felt *very* self-conscious about my appearance, but then, I decided, OK, you've felt that, now, let's think about your positives. Look how far you've come, you've become successful in your painting and writing. Besides, you're not giving the other people in the gym a chance. They're humans too. Maybe they don't care how much weight you can lift or how "unmuscular" you are.

I felt very welcome as I entered the gym the first day. Everyone was cordial, friendly and non-judgmental. Joe, the manager, couldn't have been nicer or more understanding. "Would you like to consider a private trainer? Most people do."

"*Most*?" I asked. "You mean lots of people use personal trainers?"

"Yes, they do, because otherwise they may try to use too many pounds of weights, or work the weights incorrectly. But, more importantly, your trainer will keep you disciplined. Your trainer will keep you on the program, remind you of your appointments, and make sure you do what is in your own personal best interests."

At first, I thought he was just trying to get more of my money or maybe he felt sorry for me. I had a good friend in Atlanta, Tom, who had successfully worked with a trainer, so Joe's reasoning sounded logical. "Yes, I'd like a personal trainer." Best decision I could have made.

Two days later I returned to the gym. I felt more confident and was looking forward to the next step in my physical rebuilding and therapeutic odyssey. Joe introduced me to my personal trainer, from Montreal, who spoke in lilting English with a French accent.

"Hi, I'm Lein, your new friend, but I have a feeling you may hate me after the next hour." And then she smiled. She had a warm, beautiful smile, and a curvaceous leotard-clad figure. She owned me from that moment. She had more muscles all over her body than I knew even existed. And on her they were fabulous.

For the next 24 weeks, Lein and I worked together on some of the most punishing equipment there is. My legs got stronger, my arms got larger, and my cardiovascular capabilities grew exponentially. Additionally, my eye-hand/arm coordination steadily improved, I could walk longer distances without tiring as much, and, somehow, my left-sided neglect began to improve. My motor skills have also gotten a lot better. And I am told that not only was I increasing my lean muscle mass, but I was also improving and increasing my bone mass, bone density and red bone marrow. Someone said to me, "The more Lein works you to exhaustion, the less pretty she becomes." Didn't happen.

As a secondary benefit, as I began to *feel* better, I grew steadily in self-confidence and self-esteem. I found I could actually joke with my fellow "weight lifters" whose muscles were magnificent and enormous. I would exclaim to a man with huge arms, shoulder and legs, "Remember, I *loaned* you those muscles, those shoulders, those legs. You have to return them to me. I can't go through life with these!"

As I proceeded through this physical training, I became aware that I must urge others in my age group, especially those who have survived stroke, to overcome the initial reluctance and intimidation, and venture forward to a gym. Cardiovascular improvements are achieved by riding the bicycles — it builds stamina and strengthens the heart. The treadmill and steps are not easy for someone who has difficulty walking.

In addition, there are other significant benefits: I found that virtually everyone at the gym is friendly, willing to help, understanding, and not at all in the "comparison syndrome." No one yet has sought to impress others, at least I haven't noticed. Another benefit is that the health food café has creatively improved my diet. I have lost a few pounds, eat more protein and less carbohydrates and I watch my diet like never before. And I have become leaner and stronger.

I have worked side by side with teenagers and men and women over 70 years of age. It's been a fabulous experience. Lein and her associate trainers, Teresa and Richard, have worked me on the weight machines, on the floor mats with stretching exercises, and even exercised me in the swimming pool.

These experiences were all new to me. I was never one to "go to the gym." I thought working 10-12 hours a day at the office and playing golf once a week were enough. They're not. And, I've come to realize that just because I had a brain injury, *I am not immune to any malady* and must take good care of my health. One can fall into the trap of deluding oneself that a terrible stroke somehow eliminates the possibility of some other catastrophic disease or injury. It simply isn't so, and from my view as one who has "been there," prevention is a whole lot better that the experience of going through it all over again, even if it's in a different form.

As every stroke survivor should be aware, there are continuing physical and emotional impairments that can and should be addressed with post-stroke therapies.

I have certainly benefited by involving myself in fitness and strengthening programs at the local gym. Exercise by stretching, bicycle riding or simply walking briskly as much as possible each day reduces stress while improving one's condition and muscle tone.

Before I began my exercise and strengthening program, my left leg had atrophied to about 60% of my right leg. The same was true of my left arm compared to my right arm. I was stunned that my right limbs could lift up to ten times the weight as my left limbs. However, the improvements as a result of my conditioning and strengthening program have been profound. They are nearly the same in size today, and both are a lot firmer.

I have also found that I have made many new friends. As I associate with these energetic, attractive people who are full of positive thoughts and conversations, my own energy level and positive attitudes have skyrocketed. My physical capabilities are greater, my stamina has increased, my cholesterol levels are down and my pulse rates have improved dramatically.

But a word of caution: it is true, as Rebecca has cautioned me many times, that strenuously lifting weights and straining body strengthening exercises can increase "muscle tone." In my case, I found that by concentrating on building my body strength, I increased muscle mass and tone, which actually distorted my muscle coordination. This causes short-term difficulty in walking, sometimes to the point where my body will twist, overwork my trunk muscles, and cause my legs to cramp and get very sore.

Physically, I have noticed a marked reduction in my spasticity, a better sense of balance and greatly improved posture. Stroke survivors, as a result of loss of muscle tone, tend to bend over or stoop as we stand and walk. I noticed that was my tendency. I was very conscious of my appearance, reminded by my therapist and professional trainer at the gym to "lift your head, don't look down, straighten your back, extend your left leg." I now can walk and stand so much more naturally, and I am not straining every minute.

Performing aerobic exercises, whatever the amount, will improve one's muscle tone, capabilities and attitude. Stroke survivors should respond to the admonitions of the American Stroke Association and the National Stroke Association to retain personal trainers and/or physical therapists and begin a stroke fitness and strengthening program. It should improve your ability to walk, move about, control your balance and will lift one's energy level and spirits.

I have been told "90% of your improvement will occur in the first twelve months." While hearing that bit of news may be uplifting during the first, second or third month, by the time I was in my tenth or eleventh month, I was getting depressed because I knew I was a long way from where I hoped to be. Stroke survivors can improve significantly for years and years with repetitive therapy that teaches adjacent brain cells to perform the activities formerly done by the now dead cells. For severe stroke survivors, that "90% in the first year" statement turned out to be a myth. Don't believe it.

I have seen results in myself during the past six years that I would have believed very unlikely theretofore. I am much better able to stabilize and balance my body. My "drop foot" happens when I tire, but it has become less of a problem. My left hand, gratefully, is more often than not by my side and no longer in my crotch. New research findings are very encouraging to stroke survivors. I am also aware that I continue to learn and improve as I go forward, and I certainly will never stop trying or stop my therapy. It's like driving across the country and putting your car in "cruise control." Improving my health, capabilities, and quality of life are paramount.

My life is very different and more limited than it was before my stroke, yet I can honestly say that it is a life that is indeed better in so many ways. My values and priorities are more sound, and while I continue my therapeutic odyssey, it has become a welcomed part of my life. Everyone in my world is supportive, and I look forward to each day. Enjoying my quality of life and my relationships with others is an integral part of my daily life. My improvement over these past years has surely been slow and steady, but positive and remarkable. I have succeeded in reaching a high degree of physical capability and emotional stability that for so long seemed beyond my hopes and dreams. I have come to a place of acceptance where I am actually enjoying an active, full and productive life. I am colors, I am words, I am prayer, I am happy.

Appendix

Incidence of Stroke

The frequency of occurrence of stroke is alarming. In the United States alone, someone has a stroke every 45 seconds and every 3 minutes someone dies from a stroke. These are astounding statistics and I believe most of us have no idea how prevalent strokes are.

Stroke is known as the number three cause of death in Americans (after heart disease and cancer). Statistically, more than an estimated 730,000 people have a new or recurrent stroke each year in the United States and nearly 160,000 of those will die from their stroke.

Stroke strikes a member of more than one family in five each year. If one assumes that from five to ten others, including family members, colleagues, and friends are significantly affected, then one can safely accept the estimate that two to five million Americans are impacted annually by new strokes.

Stroke is not only an "old person's problem." Strokes can occur in a wide range of age groups. One can be 18 or 65 years old, although the preponderance of strokes occurs in people over 65.

According to the NSA, "For each decade after age 55, the risk of stroke doubles. For adults age 65, the risk of dying from a stroke is seven times that of the general population. Two-thirds of all strokes occur in people over age 65." Thus, one-third, or as many as 40,000 strokes occur in people under age 65 per year. The over-50 population, the baby boomer generation, increased by 19 percent between 1994-2000. It is the fastest growing U.S. age group, and puts more people at higher risk for stroke every day. Stroke is a major and increasing factor in the late-life dementia that affects more than 40 percent of Americans over age 80.

Statistically, those living in the southeastern United States suffer the highest rate of stroke and the highest mortality rate from stroke in the United States. That region is aptly called the *stroke belt*. Within that area, Georgia and the Carolinas have twice the mortality rate of the entire United States and are called the *stroke buckle*. Florida, most likely due to its more senior population, is estimated to have 150,000 incidences of stroke each year.

Types of Stroke

In 1999, the National Stroke Association stated that, "A stroke or brain attack occurs when blood flow to an area of the brain is interrupted by a blocked or broken blood vessel. When a stroke occurs, it kills brain cells in the immediate area. When the brain cells die, they release chemicals that set off a chain reaction that endangers brain cells in a larger, surrounding area of brain tissue. Without prompt medical treatment, this larger area of brain cells will also die. When brain cells die, the abilities of that area of brain control are lost or impaired. Some people recover completely from less serious strokes, while others lose their lives to very severe ones."

The two major types of brain attacks are *ischemic* stroke, in which a clot blocks a blood vessel in the brain, and *hemorrhagic* stroke, in which a blood vessel in the brain ruptures.

A transient ischemic attack (TIA), sometimes called a mini-stroke, is milder than a stroke, yet, is not to be ignored. A transient ischemic attack refers to the temporary interruption of blood supply to the brain. The attack could last anywhere from a few minutes to an hour with no evidence of permanent damage. The symptoms simply go away. However, a TIA is a warning for the possibility of a future acute stroke that could result in more serious and debilitating consequences. Statistically, one-third of those who suffer TIAs will suffer an acute stroke in the future. More than 500,000 TIAs occur in the United States each year, in addition to the 730,000 strokes reported, for a total of 1.2 million.

Approximately 20% of *all* strokes are hemorrhagic. The survival rate for a hemorrhagic stroke is less than 25%. However, an ischemic stroke is typically not as severe, but has a much higher likelihood of recurrence. (There is always "good news, bad news.") I consider myself very fortunate to have survived my hemorrhagic stroke because the danger was so severe, and as reflected in these sobering statistics, I am lucky to be alive.

Effects of Stroke

Stroke is the leading cause of adult disability. According to the NSA, "Four million Americans are living with the effects of stroke. About one-third have mild impairments, another third are moderately impaired and the remainder are severely impaired." It often is so debilitating that the survivor considers himself a cripple, suffering permanent impairments and a painful, embarrassing, and dependent way of life that may not cause death, but to many, makes life so meaningless that death may be preferred. I know I felt that way for a time. As a result, many retreat from life, rarely leave the seclusion of home, and become detached from the world. This behavior re-enforces the sense of isolation, depression, and despair. It must be avoided if at all possible. In the beginning I had to force myself to go out in public, especially in that imprisoning wheelchair.

The most significant impact of stroke on the victim is the enormous emotional damage that in so many instances far exceeds the obvious physical damage. It is much deeper, more traumatic, and dramatically life changing. In an instant, a few seconds, a stroke victim can go from a productive, optimistic, ebullient personality to a sobbing, depressed, helpless person. It is one of the most emotionally painful experiences an individual can experience. The victim, friends, and family must watch almost helplessly as the stroke takes its toll.

Every neurologist or therapist will acknowledge the devastating damage to the stroke survivor's self-esteem, outlook on life, sense of purpose, and response to *every* relationship.   Every emotion is affected. Depression, frustration, anger, and loss of hope take the place of optimism, patience, confidence, and the will to live a full life. The change in personality is nearly instantaneous, depending on where in the brain injury occurred, and how severe the damage.

These are the kinds of emotional effects stroke victims experience. And these stroke victims are the loved ones others must visit, encourage, try to cheer up, feed, assist, bathe, and endure during the worst initial period, a period that can last for a days, weeks, or even years. The severe stroke victim is convinced it will last the rest of his life, and somehow, he or she is convinced that he or she must learn to say "good-bye" to his or her former life. It is dead. Gone. Forever. This can be the painful reality of enduring a stroke.

Need for Public Awareness

Strokes are more prevalent and discriminate than the general population would believe, since strokes and other brain injuries have not received the media attention that other serious illnesses have gotten. Most people do not know that strokes occur in the brain. Most do not recognize the symptoms of stroke, and consequently, delay getting medical attention, which is the worst possible course of action. Certain symptoms indicate that a stroke in progress must be treated as an emergency situation and not be ignored. Permanent injury can be reduced or removed if a stroke victim gets emergency assistance. *Time is vital.*

The most current information available from the NSA states that the average American stroke patient waits more than 12 hours before going to a doctor or the emergency room. Some people are still convinced that a stroke is untreatable, and thus, become so fatalistic as to refuse to be taken to the hospital. Another misconception is the belief that sudden numbness or blurred vision is something minor that will pass. This is a grave mistake.

A friend of mine told me about her aunt who suffered a severe ischemic stroke. True to her disposition of assertiveness, the aunt ordered her elderly husband to "leave me alone, I want to lie on the floor for a while," where she had fallen. She then went to sleep. The next day, still not feeling good, she told her worried but obsequious husband to "call the doctor." But nearly twelve hours had passed. Now my friend's aunt was beyond much help, bed-ridden, and faced with a need for 24-hour care which would require the couple to use their life savings for extended care, instead of for what they had hoped would be a relatively carefree retirement. Waiting to seek treatment can surely cause a great tragedy and needless suffering, to say nothing of potential financial ruin.

The point must be driven home and emphasized strongly that one sure way to resume a relatively normal life post-stroke, and eventually enjoy your new life is to be aware of symptoms of stroke. Recognize that it *is* treatable; that time is absolutely of the essence and emergency room treatment is vital. Call 911 at once.

Symptoms

The five most common stroke symptoms as described by the NSA are:

1. Sudden numbness or weakness of the face, arm, or leg — especially on one side of the body.
2. Sudden confusion, trouble speaking, or

understanding.
3. Sudden trouble seeing in one or both eyes.
4. Sudden trouble walking, dizziness, loss of balance or coordination.
5. Sudden severe headache with no known cause.

If these symptoms occur, immediate action should be taken.

My friend Lillian, 73, suffered a stroke at breakfast in a restaurant on a Saturday morning. "I feel nauseous," she told her husband. "I feel sick." He responded with, "Then let's go home." But she couldn't get out of the restaurant booth. Her left leg wasn't responding. She got scared; wisely, he called 911.

She was experiencing many of the typical symptoms: nausea, slurred speech, tingling in her left fingers, flaccid hand and arm. Fortunately, the paramedics responded quickly and she was rushed to the hospital.

Treatment

A CT scan and MRI must be taken *immediately* to determine if an ischemic or hemorrhagic stroke has occurred. Sometimes, a CT scan alone is not enough. Demand an MRI. That way, if it is ischemic, TPA, a new drug can be injected into the vein to, in most cases, eliminate or significantly reduce permanent damage and impairment. But TPA should not be administered if someone is suffering a cerebral hemorrhage. There is only a 3-hour window of opportunity.

In Lillian's case, the doctors couldn't determine from the CT scan which type of stroke she had and waited until Sunday to have an MRI. Regrettably, it was too late to administer TPA. Neurologists can't stress too strongly that decisions must be made quickly to save the stroke patient from the terrible after effects of stroke.

Prevention

Stroke prevention is possible in most cases. Among those risks that *are* modifiable are:
1. smoking- the most powerful modifiable stroke risk factor
2. hypertension
3. lack of awareness of stroke symptoms
4. excessive alcohol consumption
5. lack of exercise
6. high cholesterol
7. diet / lifestyle

Risk factors that are *not* modifiable, and should be considered as early warnings to alert potential victims of stroke, are:
1. family history of diabetes, heart disease, or stroke
2. race
3. genetics
4. gender

Stroke Organizations

The two stroke associations, the National Stroke Association (NSA) and the American Stroke Association (ASA), are both marvelous and most helpful. They not only support research and publish statistical data and new findings, but also promote support groups and sponsor education and screening programs to increase public awareness. The ASA maintains a National Stroke Registry of over 150,000 stroke survivors. They have a Stroke Family "Warmline" phone number at 1-800-553-6321. They publish <u>Be Stroke Smart</u>. The NSA also has a 1-800-STROKES hotline phone number and publishes <u>Stroke Connections Magazine</u>. Because of the NSA's influence, Congress declared May as National Stroke Awareness Month.

For additional copies
contact

The Cedars Group
P.O.Box 201
Delray Beach, Florida
33447

Fax (561)243-6344